RUNNER'S WORLD
GUIDE TO
INJURY PREVENTION

RUNNER'S WORLD® GUIDE TO
INJURY PREVENTION

HOW TO IDENTIFY PROBLEMS, SPEED HEALING, AND RUN PAIN-FREE

DAGNY SCOTT BARRIOS

RODALE

Notice

The information in this book is meant to supplement, not replace, proper exercise training. All forms of exercise pose some inherent risks. The editors and publisher advise readers to take full responsibility for their safety and know their limits. Before practicing the exercises in this book, be sure that your equipment is well-maintained, and do not take risks beyond your level of experience, aptitude, training, and fitness. The exercise and dietary advice in this book is not intended as a substitute for any exercise routine or treatment or dietary regimen that may have been prescribed by your doctor. As with all exercise and dietary programs, you should get your doctor's approval before beginning.

Mention of specific companies, organizations, or authorities in this book does not imply endorsement by the publisher, nor does mention of specific companies, organizations, or authorities imply that they endorse this book.

Internet addresses and telephone numbers given in this book were accurate at the time it went to press.

Runner's World is a registered trademark of Rodale Inc.

Printed in the United States of America
Rodale Inc. makes every effort to use acid-free ∞, recycled paper ♻.

Illustrations by Karen Kuchar
Photographs by Mitch Mandel/Rodale Images

Book design by Drew Frantzen

Library of Congress Cataloging-in-Publication Data

Barrios, Dagny Scott.
    Runner's world guide to injury prevention : how to identify problems, speed healing, and run pain-free / Dagny Scott Barrios.
        p.   cm.
    Includes index.
    ISBN 1–57954–971–3 paperback
    1. Running—Physiological aspects.   2. Running injuries—Prevention.   3. Running injuries—Treatment.   I. Title.
    RC1220.R8B37   2004
    617.1'027—dc22   2004017047

Distributed to the trade by Holtzbrinck Publishers

4   6   8   10   9   7   5   paperback

Visit us on the Web at www.rodalestore.com or at www.runnersworld.com, or call us toll-free at (800) 848-4735.

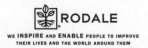

WE INSPIRE AND ENABLE PEOPLE TO IMPROVE
THEIR LIVES AND THE WORLD AROUND THEM

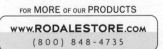

FOR MORE OF OUR PRODUCTS
WWW.RODALESTORE.COM
(800) 848-4735

For every runner who ever struggled through an injury—
which is to say, pretty much all of us

CONTENTS

ACKNOWLEDGMENTS

A heartfelt thank-you to all the running professionals who took their time to help with this book. Tim Hilden and Neil Henderson of the Boulder Center for Sports Medicine truly have the best interest of runners at heart. I thank them for agreeing to provide the expertise behind the strength and stretching portions of the book. Thanks also to Mark Plaatjes, Lewis G. Maharam, Paul Thompson, Jordan D. Metzl, Stephen Rice, Christine Wells, Margaret Karg, Matthew Callison, Yun-Tao Ma, Cynthia Ribeiro, Walter Bortz, John Cavanaugh, Bruce Wilk, Larry Grollman, Deborah Lee Greenslit, Jane Welzel, Rodger Kram, Michael Sachs, Christine Epplett, and Irene McClay Davis for being so graciously forthcoming with information, assistance, and advice. I am especially grateful to Philip Stull and Thomas Shonka, who served as arbiters on medical issues.

The wonderful team at *Runner's World* and Rodale Books ensured that this work would be as helpful to runners as possible. Thank you to copy editor Jean Rogers and project editor Kathy Dvorsky for managing the important details. As ever, a huge thank-you to Leah Flickinger for her excellent editor's eye and touch.

The runners in my life deserve special thanks: My husband, Arturo, and my training partners, Sarah Krakoff and Karen Franklin, have, once again, patiently and supportively listened to endless miles' worth of my birthing a book. Finally, thank you to my daughter, Bianca, for waiting patiently while "Mommy types."

INTRODUCTION

Injuries. I've had my share. Let's review the damage.

1994: Iliotibial band syndrome. Caught the competitive bug and bumped up my mileage recklessly like a true zealot. It was my first major injury requiring—yikes!—time off. Depression set in. Let's just say I wasn't pleasant to be around.

1996: Plantar fasciitis. The pain in my heel gets so bad that I can barely walk to work, much less run. I lose half a year of training, not to mention plenty of enthusiasm. Finally, a second pair of customized orthotics and a night splint save the day, and I'm back in business.

1997: Achilles tendinitis. Completely avoidable and utterly idiotic. But I'm training as hard as I ever have and running personal records in my thirties, so of course time off isn't even a consideration. Eventually, I don't have a choice, as my tendon is doubled in size and raw to the touch. Okay, time for a break.

1998: Stress fracture. No warning signs for this one—a metatarsal bone just had enough of hard training. Tests showed no lacy, aging bones, so nutrition wasn't the issue. However, subsequent x-rays also revealed a cracked sesamoid bone in my other foot. No wonder that's been hurting for, oh, say, 6 months or so.

Okay, you get the point. I won't even bother mentioning the high school or college years. Or the little everyday strains and niggling pains. These are just the highlights of my adult competitive career, the injuries I can mark the years by without even looking back at my training logs.

Embarrassing? Yup. Especially now that I can see how silly and avoidable most of these injuries were. Had I taken proper measures at the onset of pain, rather than barreling heedlessly forward with my training, I could have avoided a lot of agony—and ultimately taken less time off.

The good news is that I've learned from my mistakes. As my running career has matured, so has my outlook. And amazingly enough, I haven't had any debilitating injuries since that stress fracture in the late 1990s.

So what has made the difference between life as a string of injuries and running injury-free? If I had to boil it down to one thing, it would be this: paying attention to and respecting the signals my body sends, rather than ignoring them. Last summer, for example, when I felt a strain in my calf during a track workout, I immediately changed out of my racing shoes and into my heavy trainers. I tried one more 400-meter repeat. Nope, still hurt. I walked off the track without finishing the workout, went home and iced, and then took the next day off. Forty-eight hours and a little more ice later, I jogged an easy 30 minutes with no calf pain whatsoever. Years ago, I would have ignored the warning signs, "toughed out" the track workout, and suffered a full-blown muscle pull.

Of course, I still do some unwise things when my training is heating up. We all do. But as our legs acquire years of training, we learn that our body never lies. And we ignore its messages at our own peril. Running injuries are not inevitable, but they become more or less probable based on things like your levels of patience and obsession and your ability to listen to (and trust) your body.

Even with smart training and proper attention to biomechanics, nobody can guarantee that you'll never get injured. Instead, here are some good and reasonable goals for you as a runner.

- To reduce the chance of injury

- To recognize injuries early and thus minimize damage

- To treat injury appropriately and address the underlying causes

- To return to running in a manner that discourages future injury

These four goals are addressed throughout this book. Accomplish these things and, while you might not remain injury-free, you will certainly maximize your running enjoyment and keep injuries from excessively hampering your running career.

1

INJURY 101

THE BIG IMPACT OF LITTLE THINGS

A simple footstep. It's the most basic component of running. Nothing fancy about that. Running is one footstep after another. But have you ever considered just how many times you ask your body to repeat that simple act during a run? Here's an eye-opening bit of calculation.

The average distance runner covers about a yard with each step during training—anywhere from 2.5 to 4.5 feet. That translates to 1,000 to 2,000 total steps per mile, which means the runner lands on each leg 500 to 1,000 times per mile. On a typical 5-mile run, each leg will land 2,500 to 5,000 times. A runner who covers 5 miles 5 days per week, therefore, will land on each leg 650,000 to 1,300,000 times in a year. And that's just someone covering 25 miles a week. A runner training for a marathon who's regularly putting in training of 50 miles a week can easily strike the ground well over 2 million times per leg each year.

Over the course of your running life, how many times will each leg hit the ground? Well, you know how long you've been running—as they say, you do the math. It's not unusual for a longtime runner to literally take tens of millions of steps.

A little shocking, isn't it? And when viewed that way, it's no surprise that most runners will eventually suffer some injury. In fact, researchers estimate that injury strikes a quarter to half of all runners each year.

THE INJURY EQUATION

Running injuries aren't like football or skiing injuries. When we say half of all runners suffer injury each year, most are not sidelined in a cast. No, running injuries are decidedly less dramatic, if more insidious.

Many running injuries are not even noticeable when you're walking or going about other day-to-day activities. They make themselves known only when you start running. That's because in running, injury stems primarily from all those little steps—those *millions* of little steps—adding up to exert forces that at some point aggravate some link in the structural chain that makes up the running stride. Other factors that contribute to getting hurt include how the body adapts to wear and tear, the weight of each footfall, and the muscle power required to put one foot in front of the other at a good clip. Let's take a look at each factor and its role in the injury equation.

Overuse. Rodger Kram, Ph.D., has spent his life studying the human stride—along with the penguin's waddle and the elephant's stomp. A professor of kinesiology and applied physiology at the University of Colorado in Boulder, his research on biomechanics—literally, how a body moves—has led him to extensive study of distance runners.

Dr. Kram explains the phenomenon of chronic running injuries, often called "overuse" injuries, this way: "While larger forces are more likely to cause injury, most running injuries are caused by small 'wrong' forces multiplied by many repetitions."

In his class, Dr. Kram asks his students to scrape the back of their hand lightly with a fingernail. No problem. Then they are told to scrape it once hard. It hurts a bit, but no big deal. Finally, he asks them to scrape lightly again, this time repeating the action for an entire minute. At this point, "it just about starts bleeding," Dr. Kram says. Small force, many repetitions—that's an overuse injury.

A repetitive motion that rubs, tugs, or stretches in a minor way multiplied enough times can do actual damage to muscle tissue, connective tissue, even bone. Such injuries usually send advance warning of danger ahead. A pain will typically start small, eventually growing larger and louder until it demands attention. The sooner the runner recognizes the problem as something that needs to be dealt with, the better off the runner is and the more minor the injury will remain. That's why it's imperative that runners perfect the art of "listening" to their bodies.

Compensation. This is an indirect effect of repetitive aggravation. When normal running stride results in pain, a runner will eventually alter his or her stride to reduce the discomfort.

This change in gait can be conscious or not—just because you don't think you've changed your stride doesn't mean you haven't. For example, you might think that you're ignoring the pain at the base of your big toe, but in reality your body is compensating by rolling the foot in a slightly different manner to avoid putting pressure on the painful area. But any change from your normal stride can result in *new* niggling pains that can then blossom into full-blown injuries. Even an imperceptible change, just a millimeter of difference in emphasis, places greater stresses on other parts of the foot, making them susceptible to further injury.

Impact. If repetitive motion is the force behind overuse injuries, why don't people get injured just walking around? After all, people walk all day, also taking thousands of steps, sometimes covering many miles—virtually always without injury.

The reason walking generally doesn't cause injury is because it doesn't generate the same forces in and on the body as running does. Running places huge amounts of stress on the body, and those forces are a key part of the overuse injury equation. The force of impact on the ground when you're walking is equal only to your body weight. When you're running, this force multiplies by a factor of three to six times. This multiple varies depending on whether the terrain is flat or hilly (downhill running is more stressful) and on stride length (longer strides result in greater forces).

Power. Here's yet another element to add to the injury equation: The muscular contractions that occur during running are much more forceful than those that take place during walking. Running requires explosive action from the leg muscles, which in turn causes greater stress on connective tissue—the ligaments and tendons that attach muscles and bone. For example, contracting the calf muscles places a much greater strain on the Achilles tendon when running than when walking.

CAN YOU REALLY AVOID INJURY?

Add all these factors together—repetitive motion, compensation, large forces of impact, powerful muscular contraction—and you begin to understand why runners tend to get injured at some point in their career.

In fact, you might begin to wonder how you can ever *avoid* getting hurt.

Despite all those millions of steps you take as a runner, overuse injuries are not a given. Two overriding principles form the basis of preventing running injuries.

Adapt to stress gradually. Severe, sudden training changes are a risk, and all training must be based on *your individual fitness at the time.* That phrase is key. Because every runner's conditioning is different, there's no such thing as a training program that works for all runners.

A 10-mile run that would be crippling to a novice runner is a walk in the park for an experienced marathoner deep in training. By the same token, that same marathoner would be at high risk for injury if he suddenly started running fast 200-meter repeats on the track on his high-mileage legs. Likewise, a workout that might have been easy for a runner 5 years earlier could be an injury waiting to happen for the older runner who hasn't maintained a suitable fitness level.

This concept of adapting your training gradually and basing it on your current fitness is key to injury prevention and will be dealt with in more depth in chapter 2.

Fine-tune your stride and address your biomechanics. Your chances of getting hurt closely correlate with the way your feet hit the ground and the manner in which your body absorbs impact. We'll take a closer look at this concept in the rest of this chapter.

YOUR RUNNING SIGNATURE

From the time we're toddlers learning to run, each of us develops our own natural stride, our own signature of motion. Rather like fingerprints, each person's stride shares certain elements and characteristics, yet each is unique. You might have noticed that some runners' strides are so singular that you can identify the person from a distance thanks to his distinctive running style. ("There's John with that left foot kicking out to the side.")

That fact brings us to a somewhat controversial question in running circles: Should you attempt to change your stride? Before answering that, it will help to back up a bit and first ask another question. *Why* would a runner want to change his or her stride? For two reasons: 1) to gain efficiency and/or 2) to reduce the risk of injury.

The first reason has more to do with running performance than running injury but is of interest to any serious runner who wants to go faster. The efficiency of your stride directly affects your performance. The less wasted motion in your stride, the faster you go and the less tired you become. The athlete who expends the least amount of energy covering ground is at a distinct advantage.

What does this mean in practical terms? If your natural stride entails flailing your arms around and hiking your knees up to your rib cage, all that wasted motion means you're going to tire faster—and run slower.

Don't believe it? Have you ever tried to maintain your pace while taking off your T-shirt or jacket? You wind up out of breath, working much harder to go the same rate. That's because of all the wasted motion—in this case, body movements that do nothing to propel you forward.

Sloppy form requires your body to do several counterproductive

LUCK OF THE DRAW?

Some runners put in plenty of miles and never seem to get injured. Are they just lucky, or is there some magic at work? The truth is definitely a little bit of luck (think genetics) but more smarts than magic.

Runners who don't get injured tend to have impeccable biomechanics—they don't have any of the abnormalities that throw the running stride out of alignment. Most of us aren't so lucky: It's estimated that about 80 percent of runners have some mechanical inefficiency that will toss a hitch in their running stride.

But good genes alone aren't usually enough to keep you injury-free, since every body is at risk for muscle and tendon strains, stress fractures, and other injuries. That means even if you're not particularly prone to injury, you must also pay very close attention to what your body is telling you. If you feel unusual pain developing, take steps to figure out what is going on and then take appropriate action. That might mean seeing a doctor early on, changing your shoes, cutting your overall mileage, and, if you run hill workouts and track sessions, holding off on them for a week until the pain subsides.

A combination of lucky biomechanics coupled with smart training is the closest you'll get to a guarantee of injury-free running.

things at once, almost as if you're permanently trying to take off that jacket during your run—your arms reach too far up, your legs kick out to the sides, your trunk swivels back and forth. With efficient form, on the other hand, every motion propels the body in only one direction: forward. There's minimal up-and-down movement and only enough side-to-side movement of arms and trunk to balance the body. In efficient form, every element of motion helps rather than hurts your performance.

The other reason to adjust your stride is the one that's more pertinent to this book: to avoid injury or make corrections after an injury becomes evident. That's because some biomechanical stride problems are in fact an invitation to injury, Dr. Kram says.

IMPROVING YOUR BIOMECHANICS

Perfecting your running stride isn't like, say, perfecting a dive. Nobody's going to hold up a scorecard saying you got a 5.9. And you won't necessarily become the best runner on the block even if you have gorgeous running style. Perfecting your stride means finding the best stride for *you,* one that allows you to run most efficiently while minimizing motion that is liable to lead to injury.

A big part of perfecting your stride entails knowing when to leave it alone. In running, that means respecting the old adage: If it ain't broke, don't fix it. If you've never suffered any significant pains or injuries, don't make any significant changes to your stride.

But sometimes biomechanics are directly related to injury risk, particularly when anatomical abnormalities come into play. These abnormalities include leg-length discrepancies and other foot and leg problems such as flat feet or high arches, bowlegs, or knock-knees. Runners with these anatomical challenges will have strides that do indeed create the perfect recipe for our definition of an overuse injury: small "wrong" forces multiplied by many repetitions.

People with these types of inefficiencies often are the ones to say, "I just can't run—it hurts my knees too much." Or "I tried running, but it just makes me so sore." Well, sure it does. Ignored and untreated, such inefficiencies will almost certainly cause pain and eventually injury. But if recognized, many of these problems are solvable, meaning most people can run comfortably.

You can work on biomechanics in two ways, effectively changing your stride.

Change your footwear. This kind of extrinsic adjustment causes your body to adjust to an external force, in this case, the shoe or shoe supplement. Before running became one of the most popular recreational pastimes and big business to boot, there was really only one type of running shoe. It was designed simply for running, without any particular runner or runner's foot in mind. It wasn't intended to solve any problems for runners, other than offering a bit of traction and cushioning.

Shoes have come a long way, and nowadays they are sophisticated armor with which runners can fight injury. Today, shoe manufacturers offer a multitude of options, each crafted with a different type of runner in mind. There are shoes for runners who overpronate (whose feet roll inward excessively), shoes for heavy runners, shoes for runners with high arches. (For more on running shoes and how to choose the right pair for you, see chapter 3.)

In addition, numerous shoe supplements further address anatomical abnormalities—heel cups and arch lifts, cushioning and stability devices. You can even purchase customized shoe inserts crafted to address your specific biomechanical challenges. You'll know you need some biomechanical help from shoes or shoe inserts after developing discomfort or injury.

Increase your strength and flexibility. You can also alter your biomechanics from within the body, or *intrinsically*. The best way to do so is by strengthening muscles or improving flexibility under the guidance of a physical therapist or coach. (Sorry, you can't just will yourself into a different running style. It's not that simple.)

A runner's stride is the end result of numerous structural elements working together—the strength and alignment of each and every bone, muscle, tendon, and ligament in the body. And to change your stride effectively, you must address these underlying factors. To understand how this works, consider the following example. Say you run with a sloppy foot-plant in which your toes point outward, and as a result, you have knee pain. That's a problem that you can't change just by turning your feet inward slightly. What you need to address is the *reason* your feet point outward in the first place.

Now let's say that a podiatrist has discovered that the reason for the sloppy foot-plant is an imbalance in your leg musculature. To correct the

WHAT THE PROS KNOW

WHY TO LOOK IN THE MIRROR

It's awfully hard to know what your running form really looks like. You can get an idea from your reflection when you pass by a store window, or a friend might point out that one of your arms chronically droops. But for a cold, hard look at yourself, there's nothing like being videotaped. "You can videotape someone and absolutely see they are headed for an injury—and they're not aware of it," says biomechanics expert Rodger Kram, Ph.D., of the University of Colorado in Boulder.

It can be helpful, and fun, to have your running form professionally analyzed. This can be done at a sports injury center, a physical therapy clinic, or even a sports podiatrist's office.

You can watch yourself while running and have an expert point out trouble spots that might need correction. You can try to do this yourself—have a friend tape you and view the results yourself. But you might not spot every warning sign on your own. You can look for some of the more obvious form no-no's mentioned in this chapter, such as overstriding, feet pointing outward, or knees rolling in. But chances are your self-diagnosis won't be as strongly informed as a diagnosis done by a professional.

Remember, while you can't reinvent your form, you can work to strengthen and correct it. Or you might learn that you'll benefit from a different style of running shoe or shoe insert.

stride, you'll need to strengthen certain muscles and stretch others. And depending on the severity of your problem, you may need to combine these physical changes with a change in shoes to solve the problem once and for all.

Changing your gait by deliberately altering your foot placement or stride length is where controversy creeps in—and where most experts advise caution. So finally we're able to answer the question posed earlier in this chapter: It's generally accepted that to toy with one's natural running style too much can itself be an invitation to discomfort, inefficiency, difficulty running, and maybe even injury. Runners who have already become injured are the ones who might benefit from analyzing their gait and possibly working to change it.

In the end, you can change and improve your form somewhat, but you can't reinvent it, nor would you want to. (Note that here I am talking about actual conscious changes to your stride: foot placement, stride length, etc. Virtually *all* runners can benefit from making conscious corrections to their basic running *posture*.

PROPER RUNNING POSTURE

While everyone's form is unique, some elements of proper running technique are universal. Conversely, runners do some things "naturally" that drain energy, create minor aches and pains that make running uncomfortable, or even cause outright injury.

Here's a look at what constitutes good running posture, along with some form checks you can do while you're running. Never attempt to radically overhaul your technique in one decisive action, since this can lead to aches and pains on its own. Gradually make subtle shifts. One way is to spend a minute or two at the start, middle, and end of each run mentally going through a "proper-form" checklist. After this segment of the run is over, let it go. Eventually, the changes you are trying to make will become second nature.

Arms. Relax your arms and let them swing naturally at your sides. The elbow joint should create roughly a 90-degree angle,

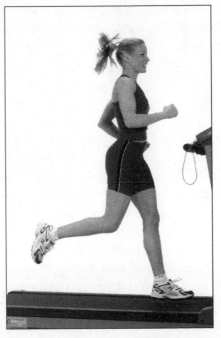

Proper form takes time to develop. Make changes gradually.

with forearm parallel to the ground. This angle should not remain rigid and robotic, however—the angle will naturally become tighter as the arm comes forward and looser as the arm swings back. Cup your hands loosely—avoid clenching your fists. Some runners make the "mistake" of letting their arms cross too far in front of their bodies, while others hold them to a rigid track at their sides. Optimal form allows for some cross-body motion as the arm swings forward.

Form check: Imagine a line down the middle of your body; be sure your hands are not swinging past and crossing this line.

Legs. Most beginning runners trot along at a shuffle during which their feet barely leave the ground. This does not enable the legs to generate much power and is typically a function of underdeveloped muscles. As you gain fitness, you'll naturally develop more leg lift. But as a distance runner, you'll never need to be pumping your legs high in the air like a sprinter. A few inches off the ground does the job.

Form check: Think about trying to cover ground in a forward direction, not vertically. Be sure you're not bounding up and down, and conversely, try not to let your feet scrape on the ground.

Feet. The feet are one area where more serious biomechanical difficulties often manifest themselves. You may need help from shoes or orthotic inserts. (For more on this, see chapter 3.)

The most natural foot strike when running distance is to land first on the outer rear portion of the heel and then let the foot roll forward and inward until pushoff from the forefoot. (A minority of runners will naturally land on their midfoot.) Avoid landing on the front of your foot. This is a classic mistake that often stems from misguided childhood gym-class instruction on sprinting. If you land on your toes, surely you're already wondering why running hurts so much and how people can possibly run as far as they do.

Form check: To learn a more natural foot strike, try walking fast and then transitioning into a shuffle-jog. Let your foot go through its natural heel-toe motion as your walk becomes a jog. As you pick up speed, notice how this heel-toe motion becomes one blended movement. Feet should ideally also be pointing straight ahead, not out to the side or inward. If your natural foot strike is "wrong"—feet pointing somewhere other than forward, weight coming down on the inside of your foot—then you're a prime candidate for corrective footwear.

Trunk, neck, and head. Your body should create a straight line from hips to head. Bending forward at the waist is a natural reaction when fatigue sets in on a run, but this can cause back strain and greatly reduces running efficiency. Likewise, a neck cocked forward is invitation to neck strain and headache.

Form check: Envision a hook dangling slightly ahead of you. Pretend that hook is attached to the *back* of your shirt collar and gently tugging you upright. A slight forward lean is okay, even preferred, but that lean should come all the way from your ankles on up in a straight line—not from a bend at your waist or your neck. Focusing your eyes several yards ahead on the road or trail can help keep your head upright and aligned with your spine. Because slouching is often the result of weak core muscles, all runners are advised to strengthen the muscles of the abdomen and back. (For more on strengthening, see chapter 5.)

STRIDE LENGTH: FINDING THE SWEET SPOT

The length of your stride is directly related to both your performance and your likelihood of sustaining injury. Short strides are generally safe—they generate less force and therefore result in less impact. But they are also "energy expensive," which means they require more steps to propel the body forward, which is less conducive to running fast or running far. Long strides are more efficient, but only up to a point, beyond which they too can waste energy. Treadmill tests (performed by Dr. Kram and many others) have shown that longer strides result in increased ground (impact) forces, which in turn can lead to injury.

The ideal stride is somewhere between short and long. "You're looking for that sweet spot that's the trade-off," he says. And fortunately, the body usually does a good job of "self-optimizing," or naturally settling into a stride that is most efficient. In an experiment, Dr. Kram asked subjects to run backward. Running backward is not something our bodies are accustomed to doing and therefore requires the body to create a "stride" from scratch. "Right away, people figured out the optimal way to do this," he says. They expended the least amount of energy in exchange for the greatest performance returns.

What is your optimal stride length? It's different for every runner, and it also changes depending on how fast the runner is going. But generally speaking, optimal foot placement for the lead leg is just slightly ahead of, or under, your center of gravity. That means your foot should fall just behind or under your knee; if the front leg reaches out excessively ahead, the braking action upon foot placement creates excessive force.

But runners don't always run with their optimal stride. Fatigue is the main reason runners fall out of their natural, optimal rhythm and into less graceful form. (Another reason is uphill or downhill terrain; still another is soreness the day after a hard workout.) Fatigue causes tired runners to look for ways to keep up the pace despite failing muscles and slowing turnover.

Picture a runner at the start of a race and that same runner as she approaches the finish line. Classic "tired-runner" form typically involves shoulders hunched up in strain, midsection collapsed forward at the waist, and legs reaching out in longer and longer strides in an increasingly frustrated attempt to cover ground quickly. It doesn't look pretty, but it's also not going to hurt you—except possibly for that increasing stride length.

Most runners will show signs of form deterioration on virtually any run, even easy distance. Think about how you feel at the beginning of a typical 5-mile run versus how you feel at the end; even if it's not noticeable to you, your form will have changed during the run—and not for the better. "Your turnover slows, so you compensate by taking longer strides," Dr. Kram explains. If you will yourself to keep up your pace, you wind up overstriding to meet that goal. "So now you're not only tired and weak, but you're hitting the ground harder," Dr. Kram says. The result? A greater chance of injury.

So, if running past the point of fatigue can be dangerous, how do you improve as a runner? It's a basic tenet of training that in order to improve, a runner must train around the edges of her ability: Both the cardiovascular and muscular systems are strengthened by stressing them slightly, then letting them recover, then doing it again and again.

The key is moderation. Dr. Kram calls it the razor's edge. "You must push yourself in order to get better, but if you push too far in fatigue, you are running in a way that predisposes you to injury."

What does it all mean to you? Your goal is to recognize when you're getting tired on a run or in a workout. When you are tired, actively work to keep your form (including your stride) under control—it's harder to do but more important than ever. Slow your pace if necessary when you're on

Review your mental checklist. At the beginning, middle, and end of every run, mentally go through a checklist of proper running posture and make subtle adjustments to your running style.

Watch yourself. Have yourself videotaped while running on a treadmill to find inefficiencies and see if your stride length needs adjusting. Get a professional evaluation or look yourself for some of the posture and form checks mentioned in this chapter.

Be aware of fatigue. Especially on very long or intense running efforts, consider cutting your workout short when you are clearly laboring to maintain a consistent pace.

Reduce impact. When possible, run harder workouts such as tempo runs on a soft surface—trail, cinder path—in order to minimize ground forces.

a distance run; cut short your interval workout if you're getting too tired to maintain proper form. Physical and mental control both play a role. It helps to keep your mind engaged by mentally ticking off a checklist of proper form elements, then making adjustments so that your body stays in form.

2

THE LAWS OF INJURY

HOW TO TRAIN PROPERLY

I f overuse leads to injury, it follows that proper use encourages healthy, trouble-free running. All those thousands of steps you take each time you run matter, but even more important is how you put all those steps together in your overall training program.

Each step is not equal to every other. Some training is smart, some foolish. Some steps will help maintain your health and fitness, and others will injure you.

In this chapter, we'll take a look at the major training-induced causes of injury and what you can do to avoid them.

THE UNDERLYING PRINCIPLE OF PROPER TRAINING

Train properly and you'll be able to run faster and farther. Train incorrectly and you'll break down instead, running slower and fewer miles—and perhaps even not running at all if you become injured.

The difference between the two scenarios lies in an equation of miles, speed, terrain, recovery, shoes, and many more minor points. To make it even more complicated, no singular equation works for every runner. We each start at different levels of fitness, we each have unique bodies, and we each have our own strengths and weaknesses. Still, we all must follow the same rules of training. One guiding principle underlies almost all aspects of the proper training equation—that of stress and recovery. *In order to get fitter, you must stress your body. But in order to reap the gains of that stress, you must then allow your body to recover.*

Proper training involves finding the balance between enough stress (running) to strengthen your body's systems and enough recovery (rest, slow jogging, or cross-training) to assimilate those gains. Each of these elements without the other is useless for gaining fitness.

In order to understand this concept, it helps to think of it in extreme terms. Let's say you decided to start running and ran as hard and fast as you could every day.

The first day, fresh and rested, you'd probably feel pretty good.

The next day, you'd probably feel somewhat sore but could probably push through that for a decent run.

By the third day, your legs would be feeling leaden and achy.

By the fourth day, you'd barely be able to run.

And by the fifth day, it's a pretty good bet you'd be injured, tendons tweaked, muscles strained.

What went wrong? No recovery, of course. In our hypothetical situation, you were asking your body to perform at its peak day after day, a physical impossibility.

Most runners aren't that foolish about their training. But we all can be surprisingly ignorant or overly enthusiastic at times, creating milder or unintended versions of the above scenario. For example, we'll jump into a new training group and start running 40 minutes, five times a week when we'd been running only a half hour two or three times a week. Or we'll decide to run a race with a friend and start doing both track workouts and hill workouts when we'd been doing neither. Or we'll skip running during a 2-week vacation and then return to our daily run as if we'd never taken a break.

These all are examples of improper training, because the stress-recovery equation is out of balance.

HOW YOUR BODY ADAPTS TO STRESS

How the body adapts to training and gradually becomes conditioned is a complicated and wondrous process. When you stress your body during a run, you actually wreak havoc on a microscopic level. Running, in fact, injures the body. And if you could get inside your cells after a run, you'd be shocked at the violence: tiny rips and tears marring your muscle fibers; tendons and ligaments traumatized by microtears and tugs; your glycogen gas tank, which provides fuel for the muscles, depleted and sitting near empty.

Of course, you can't see any of this evidence, but you can feel it—in the form of the familiar general muscle soreness and joint pain that sets in the day after a run.

Only time and rest can undo this damage. Given sufficient recovery time, the body heals its muscle fibers and replenishes its glycogen stores. The process generally requires about 2 days. If it takes longer than that, it's likely you overdid it. When the healing is complete, something amazing has occurred: The body is now stronger than it was before and able to handle greater stress, which is to say more running.

Repeat this process enough times and you experience a "training effect" or "supercompensation." Muscles, joints, bones, tendons, and ligaments all grow stronger and able to withstand more stress. Call it what you will; in layman's terms, it means you're getting in shape.

But when you don't rest your body after a run, the damage does not heal. Glycogen stores do not rebuild. That means that when you run too hard, too much, or too often, you place even greater strain on the remaining, properly functioning fibers in the body. Perhaps you've felt this before: The minor and acceptable aches and pains grow sharper and more intense. At this point, more fibers are being torn than are being repaired, and you've stressed some particular spot to the point where it can no longer function properly. In short, you're injured.

So simple! So easy to avoid! Except that it's not. There's no clear dividing line between the acceptable soreness that comes with proper training and the unacceptable pain of outright injury. Unlike a car, you don't have a red "check engine" signal that lights up when injury is imminent. Instead, it's a slippery slope, soreness leading to aggravation leading to a limp-inducing ouch.

Three principles can separate good stress (resulting in strength) from injury (resulting in debilitation).

1) Listen to your body.

2) Follow an intelligent training program.

3) And most of all, allow proper recovery time.

As you become more familiar with the amount of healthy stress your own body can handle and learn how much recovery you need, you'll find that injuries are easier to avoid.

Remember though, that getting in shape is a long-term proposition with no shortcuts. You cannot rush the stress and recovery process. The penalty for doing so is injury, which is what you're trying to avoid. If you overstress your body by running 10 miles instead of 5, you won't become twice as strong or twice as fast. You might be twice as sore, though. And you might not recover in time for your next run.

Now that you understand the stress-recovery principle of training, you can more fully understand the underlying causes of injury. To prevent injuries, follow these Five Laws of Preventing Injury. By now you won't be surprised to learn that these laws of prevention are really laws of training.

LAW NUMBER ONE:
INCREASE MILEAGE GRADUALLY

Increasing mileage is goal number one for beginners. Not surprisingly, it's also a leading cause of injury. A sudden jump in mileage clearly violates the stress-recovery principle, not allowing the body adequate rest to recover from the greater number of running steps you are taking. But it's not just beginners who fall prey to the too-much-too-fast mind-set. Experienced runners returning from injury can also increase their mileage too fast, as can runners coming back from a planned training break.

What you can do. Increase mileage methodically and incrementally. A good rule of thumb for beginners is to increase by no more than 10 to 20 percent a week. So if you are running 30 minutes a day, three times a week, the next week you'd want to run about 33 to 35 minutes on those 3 days. Also, build some plateaus into your training. After increasing your mileage for 3 weeks in this manner, hold steady for a week or two before increasing again.

Following the same principle, if you want to increase your frequency to 4 days a week, you'd still only want to increase your overall time running by 10 to 20 percent. (In our scenario, that means adding 9 to 18 minutes, tops, for the week.) So clearly, you don't just add another 30-minute run to the week. Instead, you'd be best off doing four runs of

WHAT THE PROS KNOW

HOW INJURY IS CONNECTED TO PERFORMANCE

The training principles in this chapter focus on *injury prevention*, but the same rules apply when you're trying to run your fastest, too. Unfortunately, the rules often go out the window for all but the smartest competitive runners. In fact, recovery is never more important than when you're training to race.

When peak performance is the goal, runners stress their bodies to the limit. Speed workouts, increased mileage, and especially racing cause even greater trauma to the body than easy jogging. Therefore, recovery becomes even more critical. When you become so focused on training and improving that you ignore warning signs and don't give your body sufficient rest, injury will beat you to the finish line.

The best runners understand that the athlete who wins a race often is not the one who trains the hardest but the one who trains the *smartest*. Nothing will decrease your training, fitness, and overall conditioning like a full-blown injury. Serious, competitive athletes know that the best and fastest route to peak performance comes not from running foolishly beyond one's abilities but from running free of injury.

about 25 minutes, or two runs of 30 minutes and two runs of 20 minutes with some walking before and after.

If you're a veteran runner coming back from break or injury, don't make the mistake of picking up where you left off. Depending on the length of the break or the severity of the injury, determine a comfortable base volume to start from.

Don't be proud. Even experienced, competitive runners should start very gradually after a long layoff. If an injury has set you back severely, you might have to start off as if you were a beginner: Jog a minute, then walk a minute, alternating for half an hour. From here, slowly increase the jogging portions to 90 seconds, then 2 minutes.

If your layoff was for only a few weeks, you'll probably be able to start from a base of 30 minutes of jogging a day and then increase with the same 10 to 20 percent principle.

LAW NUMBER TWO:
INCREASE INTENSITY INCREMENTALLY

"People think every workout has to look like a Gatorade commercial," says Paul Kammermeier, an exercise physiologist at the Boulder Center for Sports Medicine in Colorado. It's consistency first, not intensity that leads to fitness, he explains. If you do TV commercial—worthy workouts every day, you're more susceptible to overtraining syndrome and injury.

Faster steps place greater strain on the body than slower steps. Muscles work harder and suffer more damage, joints absorb greater impact, your body expends more energy overall. So it's pretty obvious that you shouldn't start doing hard interval workouts three times a week if your workouts have consisted only of easy jogs.

Beyond the obvious, also pay attention to "hidden" intensity in your training. Hilly runs are harder on your body than flat ones, since down-hill running exerts tremendous shock on the legs. Tempo runs are more intense than easy runs. Races count as intense runs as well.

What you can do. Introduce intensity into your running regimen gradually. A gentle way to do so for beginners is with unstructured speedplay: In the middle of your distance run, pick up the pace slightly for short durations, then return to your regular pace.

A general rule of thumb is that intense workouts—hills, track, and tempo runs—should make up no more than 20 percent of your training. So if you're running 40 miles a week as an experienced runner, you might be doing a total of 3 miles of repeats on the track on one day and a 5-mile tempo run on another day, totaling 8 miles of harder, faster running.

And keep track of your *overall* intensity equation to beware of all the places in which you are stressing your body. Never add more than one intense element into your training at a time. For example, if you are just starting to do hill workouts once a week, wait another 2 or 3 weeks before adding track or tempo workouts into the weekly mix. Or, if you ran a race on Sunday, don't do your normal track workout on Tuesday; do something less strenuous instead.

Likewise, increase the intensity of each type of workout gradually. For example, let's say your tempo run is normally 2 miles in duration, but now you want to start training for a marathon. Don't bump up the length of the tempo run to 4 or 5 miles right away. Instead, increase it to 3 miles for a few weeks, then 4 miles for a few weeks after that.

LAW NUMBER THREE:
INCREASE MILEAGE AND INTENSITY SEPARATELY

As you gain fitness, you'll naturally want to run longer—or faster. That's great. Just don't plan on doing both at the same time. Increased mileage and speed place more stress on your body. And each requires greater recovery. So it goes without saying that if you add both into your training program at the same time, you risk injury.

What you can do. Runners generally should increase their mileage before increasing their speed. Especially if you're a novice, focus first on building mileage. Maximize the gains you make from simple distance runs before adding faster workouts into the mix. This is sometimes called "building a base." By building a base of solid mileage at a slower, steady speed, you prepare your body to handle the stresses of faster workouts to come.

A good goal is to be able to run 30 minutes four times a week. Once beginners have met this milestone, they can eventually build to a fifth day of running. The next step is to gradually extend one of the runs from 30 to 60 minutes. This 1-hour run will become the basis of longer runs should you want to run races longer than a 5-K. Once you can run this schedule comfortably for several weeks, you are ready to add a more intense workout of hills or intervals.

Experienced runners must follow the same principle. Generally speaking, add mileage early in the year. Once mileage is at a sufficient level, you can add faster workouts. For example, let's say you ran a major goal race such as a half-marathon or marathon late in the fall. You might have rested for much of the month of December as a break. Come January, the focus would be on distance, building mileage to reestablish a solid base. Sometime in February or March, you would begin adding some fartlek (running segments that alternate faster stretches with slower, recovery stretches) or hill workouts once a week. By April, you'd be ready to hit the track, adding a day of speedwork. With this gradual approach, you won't shock your body with too much stress.

LAW NUMBER FOUR:
ALTERNATE HARD EFFORTS WITH REST

Again, this follows clearly and directly from our stress-recovery principle. You must allow your body to recover from hard running with outright rest or a recovery run.

Most coaches' running schedules adhere to the hard-easy principle. Look in any training book and you'll find that programs rarely call for back-to-back hard efforts. Instead, intense training days are spaced out over the course of the week, with slow jogging days or days off in between.

What you can do. For novice runners, every run is hard, because the unconditioned body is adapting to all the new stresses of running. So the best running program for complete beginners is one that alternates training days and rest days, essentially running only every other day for the first few weeks—meaning 3 or 4 days a week maximum. Once you are comfortable at this frequency and can jog pain-free for 30 minutes three or four times a week, you can add another day of running to the schedule.

Veteran runners still need to rest between hard efforts. Intense running—a race, say, or a track workout—produces more inflammation and microtears in the muscles than easy jogging. Recovery after these days is essential. But because an experienced runner's body is better conditioned, these runners can accomplish this recovery with a slow, easy jogging day that doesn't tax the system to a great degree.

When training hard, monitor your body carefully and be flexible. Sometimes the one scheduled rest day is not enough, and it's helpful to be willing to change your training calendar when necessary. For example, let's say you ran a track workout Tuesday and then jogged slowly on Wednesday. Now it's Thursday, and you have a tempo run planned. But you feel sore during your warm-up, and a pain in your calf starts growing as you begin your tempo run. A wise runner would slow down and just jog easily, perhaps trying the tempo run again on Friday, after another recovery day.

Only very experienced competitive runners should attempt to run intense workouts on back-to-back days. The logic behind this type of training typically is to run on "tired legs," thus simulating intense race conditions. This violates the hard-easy principle and directly increases risk of injury. No matter how fast or experienced, even these runners must listen to their bodies carefully and closely when they attempt such training. If pain develops or muscle soreness from the previous day's workout is intense, the second workout should be aborted.

LAW NUMBER FIVE:
PAY ATTENTION TO EARLY WARNINGS

We've seen that most running injuries are overuse injuries due to improper training and/or biomechanical inefficiencies. That means, in most cases, the body will send warning signals before the injury manifests itself fully: Pain in a joint. Soreness in the heel. Something not quite right that doesn't go away after a day or two but instead grows worse.

Red flags are meaningless unless you pay attention. It's up to you to heed these signs. You're the only one who knows how your body feels. Even the best coach can't determine that an injury is lying in wait. Your training partner can't know that your hamstring is screaming. The responsibility for listening to your body and then acting intelligently lies squarely with you.

What you can do. Expect a certain amount of muscle soreness when you begin running or amplify the intensity of your training. That type of general, nonlocalized pain typically diminishes in a few days and is not cause for concern.

On the other hand, any sharp pains or joint discomfort during your run are the red flags of real injury. Deal with this kind of pain immediately with rest or treatment. Sharp muscular pains can signify pulls or strains. Pain in the foot, back, knee, or other joints is also likely a sign of injury.

If pain is sudden or becomes worse during a run, first slow down and see if the pain abates. If not, stop running and walk back. Either way, finish the run in as short a distance as possible. It's fine to try running the next day, but if the pain resumes, it's time to see a physical therapist or sports medicine physician. (For more on how to proceed when you are injured, see chapter 8.)

Pay attention to even seemingly minor discomforts. It's much easier to apply ice and rest a day or two for a minor strain than to recover from a torn muscle. It's faster and cheaper to go to the podiatrist and get your feet analyzed when pain is minor than to rehabilitate painful runner's knee and then get fitted for orthotics. Even a blister should be addressed and treated properly, since running on a blister can lead to compensation in the stride that can in turn lead to other problems.

IT'S THE LITTLE THINGS THAT COUNT

We've addressed the prime injury risk factors and what you can do to minimize them with smart training. But many other factors can also affect a runner's health. Paying attention to the following details will ensure that you're running smart and doing everything possible to avoid injury.

Take the time to warm up gradually every time you run. Muscles and connective tissue that have been at rest and are "cold" are more prone to injury. A proper warm-up limbers the body and coaxes bloodflow to the tissues that do the hard work of running, making pulls and strains less likely.

While most runners recognize the importance of warming up before races or track workouts, these same runners often bolt off at full speed on regular, daily runs. "Going too fast, too hard, too early on a run is one of the biggest mistakes runners make," says Bruce Wilk, a longtime runner who sees plenty of injured athletes at Orthopedic Rehabilitation Specialists, his Miami-area physical therapy practice, and at The Runner's High, the running store he owns there.

The runner might not feel any pain immediately, but inflammation and tissue failure become evident a day or two later. "What begins as an unidentified small injury then magnifies over weeks," Wilk says. "It can set a whole cycle in motion." This particular injury spark is avoidable with proper warm-up.

Improper warm-up can also cause injury, though. "Stretching is not warming up," Wilk points out. "Going easy before going hard is warming up." Stretching a cold muscle can cause as much—or more—damage as running hard.

A proper warm-up consists of:

• Extremely slow jogging or walking for 5 minutes

• Then jogging slightly slower than your typical pace for a few more minutes

• Stretching gently now that your blood is moving

• If you're racing or doing a faster workout, now's the time to run some strides at the intensity of your desired effort

• Or, if your workout is just a steady run, simply resume running and gradually work into your desired pace

Ideally, use this warm-up process on every run, but it's more important at some times than others. In cold weather, the warm-up is critical because you're battling external conditions that tighten the body's soft tissues, making them more prone to injury with sudden exertion. Warming up also is more important for morning runners, who crawl out of bed and hit the trails within minutes of waking. These runners literally must get their blood moving and loosen their limbs before hitting full stride; runners who train in the afternoon or evening have a whole day of walking around, bending, and stretching that serves to limber the body without a formal warm-up.

Drink enough. Hydration is important not only in regulating body temperature and excreting toxins but also for preventing injury. That's because a dehydrated muscle is more susceptible to strains and tears. (For more on proper hydration and its link to heat illness, see chapter 7.)

Eat right and take a daily vitamin supplement. Proper nutrition directly affects the health of your bones and muscles. That means what you eat can make you either more or less likely to become injured. Protein, for example, is a must for muscle repair. Women need enough calcium to prevent stress fractures. The right balance of minerals helps prevent cramping.

Fancy diet tricks aren't necessary and, in fact, are more often harmful than helpful. The right diet for a runner is the simple, commonsense diet you've been admonished to eat for years. The bulk of a runner's diet— some 65 to 70 percent—should consist of carbohydrates from healthy, unrefined sources such as brown rice, whole wheat pasta, and fruits and vegetables. Another 15 to 20 percent of calories should consist of protein from lean meat sources, fish, soy, or legumes. The remaining calories should come from fats, heavy on the healthy nonsaturated versions— olive or soybean oil, nuts, and the like as opposed to butter or other saturated fats.

Women in particular should also make the effort to consume adequate calcium and iron. And all runners benefit from the antioxidants found in fresh fruits and vegetables. While it's always best to meet nutritional needs through proper diet, a daily multivitamin can help as insurance. Choose a supplement geared toward active men or women for a formula that best meets your particular needs, but stay away from those that exceed the recommended Daily Value of any vitamins or minerals.

Get plenty of sleep. When we talk about recovery within a running program, the principle doesn't apply only to resting your muscles. It's important to allow your entire body and all its systems to recover, and that's accomplished only with adequate deep sleep. During sleep, the body produces human growth hormone, a prime tool in the recovery and repair of damaged cells.

How much sleep you need is highly individual; some adults thrive on as few as 6 to 7 hours, while others require 8 or 9 to feel vibrant. One way to gauge whether you're getting enough sleep is whether you are able to wake up at your required hour without an alarm clock. If your alarm typically rouses you from a deep sleep, chances are you need more rest. But if your body is beginning to stir at that time, you've probably had your fill.

As you increase your training, you might notice your sleep patterns changing. Studies have shown that regular exercise makes it easier to fall asleep. And the more intense your running program is, the more sleep you'll likely need to recover from the ensuing stress to your body. (Running too close to bedtime can make it more difficult to sleep, since your body remains revved up for several hours after vigorous exercise. To ensure a good night's rest, run at least 3 or 4 hours before you plan to sleep.)

Fully rehabilitate previous injuries. Studies show that one of the best indicators of future injury is previous injury. Injury can recur because an area did not heal sufficiently before running stresses overwhelmed it again or because the area healed in a weaker, compromised form after injury.

Therefore, it's critical to let injuries fully heal before you resume a full running load. Running gently and at a reduced mileage while you heal is fine for many injuries, but hold off on the more intense running until you're entirely pain-free.

Also, address underlying causes that created the injury; the last thing you need to do is make the same mistake twice. Replace shoes, change your running schedule, see a podiatrist for orthotics—make sure you know why your injury occurred so you can make more intelligent choices in the future.

Finally, continue to address the problem area with extra love and care even when you believe your injury is behind you. The type of injury will determine exactly what kind of long-term maintenance program this entails—perhaps icing, massage, stretching, or strengthening. Ask a physician or physical therapist for an appropriate course of action.

Be flexible about your workouts. It's worth repeating: Runners who are unwilling to change their plans are asking for trouble. View your planned schedule as a guideline, but always be willing to change when your body is hinting that it could use a rest. If your schedule calls for a hill or track workout but your Achilles is a little sore, switch to flat terrain and run easy distance for a day or two. That one missed workout is no big deal; an aggravated tendon that sets you back for several weeks is a much bigger deal.

Other factors might change your plans as well. If it's cold and windy the day of a planned speed workout and the next day is supposed to be warmer, change your plan and run the hard workout on a warm day, when you won't be as susceptible to muscle strains. Of course, this might require an evaluation of the rest of the week, since you don't want to pile your hard workouts on top of each other. You'll have to use your judgment and let your body guide you. For example, running a speed or hill workout the day before a long run is fine for some experienced runners but not for novices. The novice might want to skip either the long run or the workout for the week.

Vary your terrain. Too much of any one thing is not a wise running plan. Hills are wonderful for training, for example, but if you run on them every day, you might overstress your quadriceps and Achilles tendon. Give your legs a break by running easy days on flatter trails.

Be careful, too, of running the same roads every day. Many roads have a slant, or camber, that raises one leg higher than the other and places both feet on a pronounced slant—that's an invitation to injury. Try not to run on such roads day after day.

Vary your workouts in order to balance your muscle requirements. Repeating the same workout day after day is a recipe for injury. Even with proper rest between workouts, however, it's wise to vary the stresses on your system. That means mixing up your types of runs and, for some people, also varying your sports.

Cross-training is most important for novice runners, whose bodies are still struggling to adapt to the stresses of training. When beginning a running program, plan on alternating days of running with other

WHAT YOU CAN DO

Get enough rest. By following this underlying principle of training, you can avoid many potential injuries.

Never increase mileage or intensity abruptly. And don't increase both at the same time. Pay attention to all the various sources of stress in your training and make incremental increases overall.

Heed early warning signs. Go ahead and "push through" when you're tired, but don't try to continue running through pain. Determine why the pain is occurring so that it doesn't become worse.

Take good care of yourself. Eat right, stay hydrated, get enough rest. Your body's health and fitness are the sum result of everything you put in it and do to it.

Be flexible and patient. These just might be your most important attributes when it comes to preventing injury. Runners who are impatient and rigid are setting themselves up for trouble. They're more interested in telling their bodies what to do than in listening to them.

---

workouts that stress different systems. Swimming and biking are good complements because no shock is pounding the joints and because the body is relying on different muscles. (For more on cross-training, see chapter 6.)

Experienced runners also benefit from varying the stresses on the body. This ensures that all muscles work and rest in a balanced manner. If you run every day, you can accomplish this by mixing straight track intervals with tempo runs, for example, or by alternating fartlek with hill workouts.

Run on soft surfaces. Soft surfaces generate less impact on the legs and are therefore more forgiving for runners. For this reason, trail runners suffer far fewer impact injuries than their road-running counterparts. Trails and dirt paths are beneficial for another reason, too: The uneven nature of the terrain means your feet won't land in exactly the same manner with every footstep. This variety is less likely to cause overuse injuries, and it develops balance and strength in the foot and ankle. If pavement is your most accessible running surface, make the effort to get out on dirt trails, cinder paths, or wood-chip trails at least once a week. Even a blacktop bike path is easier on the legs than a concrete sidewalk. Mix it up and choose softer surfaces whenever possible.

Take at least 1 day off a week. Some studies have shown that the overall number of a runner's consecutive training days directly correlates to the incidence of injury. So building a rest day into your schedule is an insurance policy of sorts, giving your body a break just in case some hidden strains are beginning to play out somewhere in your body. Surely, some runners are able to run every day, never taking a break or a day off. But for most runners, even the most experienced, taking 1 day off a week is good advice. The only runners who can and should be running daily are serious, competitive-caliber runners.

Take at least one break during the year. Allow your body at least 1 week of full rest during each year. Just like your 1 day off a week, this will serve as an insurance policy against hidden strains that might be building unbeknownst to you. An added bonus is that you'll get a mental break, and you'll probably return to your training rested and ready to go. Plan your break for after the completion of a marathon or other major goal race, when you'll want to rest anyway. Or schedule a break around your vacation or business travel time, when it's more of a burden than a pleasure to train.

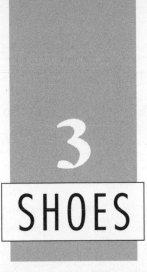

3

SHOES

THE RUNNER'S EQUIPMENT

Forget any fashion statement your running shoes might make. The most helpful way to think of running shoes is not as apparel at all but rather as serious, specialized sports equipment. "Equipment is critical in any sport—skiing, cycling, football. If your equipment gets messed up, you can get hurt," says Bruce Wilk, running shoe specialist and director of Orthopedic Rehabilitation Specialists in Miami. It's no different with running. And shoes are the primary—arguably the only—crucial piece of equipment our sport requires.

Running shoes are a safety device and performance enhancer. They hold the secret to security and comfort. They literally provide the foundation of every run. And they should never, ever be an afterthought. "Runners have to make the right choice every time they put shoes on their feet," Wilk says. "Not only in the store but also as the shoes age."

VISIT THE RIGHT STORE

When you shop for running shoes, your first stop should be a running specialty store. If there's one in your town, consider yourself lucky.

WHY RUNNING STORES RULE

Besides having the best selection and sales staff, there's another reason to visit a running store: Such stores become a community hub of information on the sport. They'll have fliers for races, coaches, and training groups. They'll sell the latest accessories, watches, hydration devices, jogging strollers, and more. The folks you meet there will know everything there is to know about running in your town, from the best doctors to visit to the best trails to run. Most running stores host group runs, and some offer seminars that are a terrific source of information. You might pick up tips from a nutritionist or learn self-massage from a professional massage therapist. Plus, you never know who'll be working behind the counter. Often these stores are owned by former running stars or are staffed by up-and-coming hopefuls in the sport.

If the nearest one is an hour or so away, get in the car and drive; it's worth the trip. To find out if there's one near you, check out the *Runner's World* magazine Web site, www.runnersworld.com.

Running stores carry a wider range of models to choose from than most general sporting goods stores. Even more important, the staff at running specialty stores are usually serious runners with years of experience in the sport who can help you figure out what type of stride you have and what type of shoe will serve you best. They also have the best understanding of the technology that underscores today's running shoes. These are things "that the average high school kid helping you at the mall can't do," says biomechanics expert Christine Epplett, who develops running shoes for New Balance in the Boston area.

You'll find a few other bonuses at running stores, too. Most running stores will let you take the shoes for a test run outside. They offer a wide range of socks, inserts, and arch supports to try on with the shoes. Some stores even have a treadmill rigged with a video camera that enables the salesperson—and you—to view you running on a television screen.

While not exactly scientific, a video can open your eyes to some of your more obvious biomechanics and help point you in the direction of the right type of shoe.

HOW RUNNING SHOES WORK

Choosing the right running shoe means choosing the shoe that's best for your body type and running program. A pair that's perfect for one runner very well could be exactly the wrong pair for another, which means that what works for your friend or training buddy won't necessarily work for you. Your goal is to figure out what type of shoe is best for your individual needs.

Before trying to choose the right shoes, it helps to understand what running shoes are designed to do. Running shoes should do the following to some degree or another.

- Cushion to protect against impact when your heel strikes the ground

- Align your foot and help to distribute force beneficially

- Protect your foot as a barrier between you and the ground

Accomplishing all these things is a complex process. When running, the foot maneuvers through a wide range of motions. The shoe must accommodate the foot throughout the whole cycle from heel strike to toe-off. In addition, each runner's foot is unique, a singular combination of high or low arch, long or short toes, wide or narrow heel, flexible or rigid ankle, and any number of other factors.

So just because all running shoes cushion and protect in some form or another doesn't mean any shoe will do. Each running shoe is designed with a particular type of body and stride in mind. The right shoe will minimize your biomechanical abnormalities and allow you to run pain-free; the wrong shoe easily can exacerbate such problems.

Shoes tend to fall into one of the following three categories.

Stability. Stability shoes are designed to control excess pronation, or inward foot rolling. They are also called "motion control" shoes. They feature rigid devices around the heel and arch. They typically are designed in a line that falls straight between the heel and toe, meaning that if you place a ruler down the middle of the sole, the center of the heel

SHOE TALK

A lot of technical talk is bandied about when discussing shoes. Here are definitions for some of the terms you'll run across in this chapter and in the store.

Pronation. The inward rolling motion the foot makes in the course of a footstep. In a normal foot strike, a runner lands on the outside of the back of the heel. The foot then rolls forward and inward until push-off occurs, typically from just inside the center of the forefoot. Pronation is natural and necessary: The sequence of movement from heel to toe distributes shock and prepares the foot for proper takeoff. However, excessive pronation—sometimes called hyper-pronation or overpronation—can create problems. When a runner pronates excessively, the foot rolls in too much, and several areas can become strained. Injury can result, including aggravation to the plantar fascia, Achilles tendon, and knee.

Supination. An outward rolling of the foot during the foot strike. It is much less common than overpronation. Supinators tend to have high, firm arches and rigid feet. The lack of pronation during foot strike can lead to pain and injury for supinators, because impact forces are not being absorbed well. Think of it as the difference between rolling with a fall and absorbing the shock of a fall suddenly.

Outsole. The outsole is the bottom layer of the shoe, the part that makes contact with the ground. It is designed with durability and traction in mind and might also house or be layered with components designed to make the shoe more stable.

Midsole. The midsole is the layer between the outsole and the

and toe fall on a straight line. They might also have other technical features, such as a flared heel, to reduce pronation. The soles of stability shoes should be fairly rigid. That means they shouldn't torque much from side to side if you twist them, and they shouldn't give much if you try to bend them.

Cushioning. Cushioning shoes offer maximum shock absorption upper body of the shoe. It provides most of the cushioning and, depending on the material, can also provide stability.

Upper. The upper is the portion of the shoe that wraps around the foot and laces on top. Typically created of a combination of leather and synthetic materials, the upper also provides important structural support.

Last. The last, or mold that the shoe is created on, determines the overall fit of the shoe—whether it conforms well to your foot or feels too wide or too narrow. When it comes to shape, shoe lasts vary among manufacturers and also among different models from the same brand. The last also refers to the type of construction inside a shoe: A *slip last* is sewn together moccasin-style at the bottom, offering flexibility; a *board last* is firmer and provides greater stability. Some shoes feature board lasting that covers the back portion of the shoe, from the heel to the midfoot; this is sometimes known as a *combination last,* and it offers a medium range of stability.

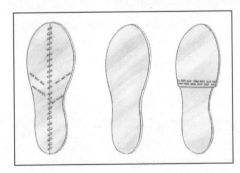

SHOE CONSTRUCTION

A slip last (left) offers flexibility; a board last (middle) provides greater stability; a combination last (right) provides both.

and are intended for supinators and underpronators. Cushioning shoes don't have stability devices to control excess pronation, since they're designed to maximize the foot's ability to flex. These shoes absorb shock with a more yielding construction (typically curved between the toes and heel) and softer materials with more give. The midsole and overall construction of a cushioning shoe is generally quite flexible: You

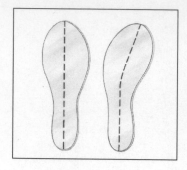

LAST SHAPES

Stability shoes (left) have a straight last and provide support for overpronators. Cushioning shoes (right) use a curved last offering maximum shock absorption for underpronators.

will likely be able to twist it in your hand from side to side and bend the toe up toward the heel.

Combination or neutral. These shoes feature some motion control but not as much as a stability shoe. They are somewhat flexible and offer a moderate degree of cushioning and shock absorption. Biomechanically efficient runners with no major history of injury are the best candidates for combination shoes.

This category breakdown is crucial for runners to understand. If you need pronation control but choose a cushioning shoe, you'll allow torque to multiply as your foot rolls unchecked through each landing. If you require cushioning but mistakenly choose a stability shoe, you will exacerbate your already rigid foot strike and the ensuing impact forces. In short, this distinction can make or break an injury. The key is knowing which category is best for you and finding the best fit within that category for your foot.

HOW TO CHOOSE YOUR SHOES

Now you're ready to focus on finding the best model of shoe for you. Several factors should go into your choice. These are the pri-mary ones.

Degree of pronation. Runners who pronate excessively should choose a stability shoe. Runners with more rigid feet who underpronate need a cushioning shoe. Efficient runners with no obvious biomechanical abnormalities should choose a combination shoe.

How do you know if you overpronate or underpronate? This is where a visit to a running specialty store helps, since the staff can examine your running style and help you make that determination. But if you're on your own, you can still make an educated decision by using the Wet

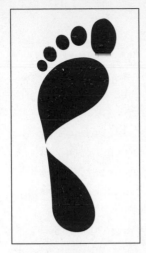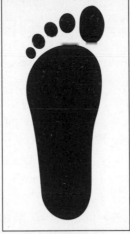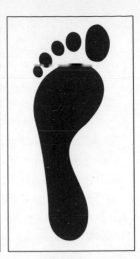

THE WET FOOTPRINT TEST

When the forefoot and heel are separated, you have a rigid foot that requires cushioning (left). When the forefoot and heel are connected and most of the arch area leaves an imprint, you have a flexible foot that pronates and requires stability (middle). When the forefoot and heel are connected by a thin slice of arch, the foot is normal and can run in combination shoes (right).

Footprint Test, which will tell you if you have flat feet or high arches. Flat feet tend to overpronate, since the arch collapses upon contact with the ground, allowing the foot to roll inward.

This test isn't infallible but should give you an idea which category you fall into. Here's how to do it: Wet your feet in a bath or tub of water. Then step on a dark towel or flat rug and take a full step, letting your feet go through their natural range of motion. Examine the footprints left behind.

Or a friend can watch you from behind as you first walk and then run. The more your foot visibly collapses inward after it strikes the ground, the greater your degree of pronation. Your friend can also watch to see if your toes point out, also typically a sign of overpronation.

Body weight. The heavier the runner, the sturdier and beefier the shoe should be. Heavy runners experience greater forces of impact, requiring more of whatever it is they need: more stability or more cushioning, depending on their foot strike. They will break down less durable, lightweight shoes quickly.

Lighter runners can get away with a lighter shoe. Smaller impact forces mean they don't break shoes down as quickly. Some heavy shoes

TRAIL SHOES

Trail shoes are a relatively new breed of shoe. Designed to perform off-road in a variety of conditions, they generally have a grippier tread, a more durable upper, a protective toe bumper, a sturdier midsole through which rocks can't be felt, and a lower overall profile (meaning they are built closer to the ground, which helps to prevent ankle twists) than road-running shoes. Beyond this, they fall into one of the three aforementioned categories: stability, cushioning, or combination.

When choosing a trail shoe, follow the same rules as for road-running shoes. Overpronators should look for a trail shoe with stability features. And while trail shoes in general have firmer construction than road shoes, underpronators still can find trail shoes with a greater degree of cushioning.

As they have evolved from the fringes of the sport, trail shoes have become increasingly specialized so that you also can match your shoe choice to the type of terrain you run. For example, if you'll be skipping from rock to rock in the mountains, look for the stickiest rubber outsole you can find. If your runs will include river crossings, choose a model that is waterproof or allows moisture to drain from the shoe. Finally, if you'll be using the shoes for a mix of road and trail, look for a model that provides adequate cushioning and does not have an excessive tread profile.

can be overkill for a light runner, not allowing enough of the foot's natural motion to occur.

Running program. Generally speaking, the more miles you run, the more technical a shoe you need. Only super-efficient runners with no biomechanical difficulties can get away with a pared-down shoe when they're running high mileage.

Based on these criteria, you should now have an idea of whether you require a stability shoe or a cushioning shoe and whether you need a heavy-duty, technical shoe or a lighter, simpler shoe.

IF THE SHOE FITS . . .

Once you've determined the general category of shoe you should be looking at, the next step is to narrow down your choices to the best one or two, and that will depend on fit.

Fit is a highly personal matter of preference. I'm always amazed at the number of runners who ask other runners which shoe they wear and recommend, as if that seal of approval means the shoe would be right for anyone. That's not how it works.

To find the shoe that fits you best, first try on numerous pairs. Grab a model (within the proper category—stability, cushioning, or neutral) from each of the major manufacturers. Forget the latest ad campaign that caught your eye. You're looking for the brand that fits your foot best. Give them all a try.

Each manufacturer's shoes will fit differently because each crafts its shoes on uniquely devised lasts. Some manufacturers are known for fitting narrow feet better—Nike and Asics, for example—some for having wider toe boxes—Saucony and Adidas. Also, New Balance is widely praised as a pioneer in offering its shoes in variable widths; now several manufacturers have followed suit.

Most of the major running shoe manufacturers design men's and women's shoes on gender-specific lasts, with the women's shoes featuring narrower heels and a longer, slimmer toe box than men's. A few women with wide feet do prefer men's models, but most feel more comfortable in women's shoes.

Once you've chosen half a dozen shoes that fall into your general cushioning or stability category, it's time to try them on. Remember to wear your running socks and leave your street-shoe socks at home. Sock thickness can change the size and fit of shoe you require. Once the shoes are on your feet, try jogging in the store to get a real sense of fit. Or better yet, get off the carpet and go outside and run a bit if the store allows it.

Keep in mind that running shoes do not need to be "broken in." If they are tight and uncomfortable at the outset, they will not get better with time, and they are the wrong shoe for you. Running shoes should feel completely appropriate from the start. The shoe that fits should offer:

Minimal slipping. Your heel should not rise out of the shoe when

A WORD ABOUT RACING SHOES

Light, streamlined, glovelike in fit, racing shoes can make every runner feel like a champion on the starting line. But when the gun goes off, are those shoes serving you well?

For a runner used to the solid, supportive ride of a Cadillac on his feet, flighty little sports-car shoes offer scant protection and should be approached with caution.

Racing shoes run the gamut from extremely lightweight slippers that provide zero support to beefier models that can serve as light-weight trainers. It's very important to match your model of racing shoe not only to your body type but also to the race and speed you'll be running.

Generally speaking, the longer the race, the sturdier a shoe you'll need. Also, the heavier you are and the more biomechanical ineffi-ciencies you have, the more support and/or cushioning you'll need in your racing shoe.

In other words, the same rules apply to racing shoes as to training shoes. Don't make the mistake of throwing the rules out the window when it comes to competition. If you're a recreational runner and put on some featherweight racers for your marathon, you're just begging for an injury. Twenty-six miles allows plenty of

you walk or run. If the shoe slips excessively, that motion can lead to blisters. The midfoot should fit snugly but not too tight. Check to see that the lacing system enables you to get the fit you want.

Extra length. When you run downhill, your foot shifts forward slightly, moving your toes farther toward the front. So even if the shoe feels fine on a flat surface, you need about half an inch between your toes and the front of the shoe.

No rubbing. Make sure the shoe does not rise too high in the ankle area. You should not feel anything rubbing on your ankle bones or Achilles tendon. There should be no tight spots anywhere on the shoe or any sharp or wrinkled material jabbing you.

time for injury to occur. Even shorter races can cause trouble, especially if you're used to more support and cushioning.

Here are some rules of thumb for choosing racing shoes.

• Look for the same qualities in your racing shoes as you require in your training shoes. If you need motion control, don't get a flexible slipper. Get a racing shoe with some structure and heel to it.

• The longer the race, the more support and/or cushioning you'll need. You might be able to get away with a pared-down shoe for a mile or 5-K, but that same shoe can cause trouble in a 10-K.

• If you wear orthotics in your training shoes, look for a racing shoe that you can insert these into. In many racing shoes, the sock liner is glued in (as opposed to training shoes, in which it's a separate, removable piece). If possible, choose a shoe with a removable liner. Otherwise, it's okay to pull out the glued-in liner and replace it with your orthotics, as long as this doesn't raise your foot so high in the shoe that your heel slips out the back.

• Replace racing shoes after fewer miles than training shoes. They are not constructed with durability in mind. For frequent competitors, a new pair of racing shoes each season might be in order. For those who race less often, plan on buying a pair every other year.

Once you've found one or two manufacturers whose shape feels right to you, you can focus on choosing more specifically from the range of models. Try on an additional shoe or two from your chosen category. Most manufacturers, for example, make a variety of stability and cushioning shoes: some for lighter runners, some for heavier; some for high-mileage competitors and some for recreational runners.

In the end, a lot comes down to trial and error. You can do all your homework and try on many models in the store, but there's nothing like experience to teach you what shoe works best. The longer you've been running, the greater a sense you'll acquire for what works for you and what doesn't.

If you buy a shoe and you realize after a few runs that it's clearly wrong—it hurts to run in or your knees or feet have suddenly started hurting—return to the store and try to exchange it. Most reputable running stores will allow you to return shoes you've worn.

Sometimes shoe problems won't be so clear-cut, but you'll notice pain or injury starting after a month or two. "It all comes down to trying the shoes out on the run," Epplett says. If this happens to you, it's a wise investment to cut your losses and try a new and different pair of shoes. After your first few purchases, you'll be better attuned to what works and what doesn't and more likely to make the right choice for your needs.

WHEN TO REPLACE YOUR SHOES

You should always replace your shoes after an injury to ensure maximum support as you heal. And whenever your training changes dramatically—you increase your mileage in preparation for a race, you end a long cycle of high mileage—you need new shoes.

As your shoes accumulate miles, they wear out on their own—midsoles compress, outsoles erode, uppers deteriorate. When this happens, shoes lose their protective ability. The materials that provide cushioning and support lose their integrity. They no longer absorb shock. They collapse rather than control. At this point, the compromised shoe is unable to do its job.

Shoes should be replaced *before* they wear out. But how do you know when a shoe is past its prime? There's no preset expiration date for shoes, especially since individual runners put wear on their shoes differently. "It will be very different for a female of 100 pounds versus a male of 250 pounds," shoe developer Epplett says.

Generally speaking, a shoe's life lasts somewhere between 300 and 500 miles. But this is just a guideline, experts caution. Here are some additional ways to gauge whether your shoes are past their prime.

Aching legs. Sometimes it's hard to tell when shoes are worn out. The only clue might be a vague achiness in your feet or legs, especially if you haven't changed your training, or a sense that you're feeling the ground under your feet a bit too much. If this is the case, but you're not sure it's because of your shoes, Epplett recommends purchasing a new pair of shoes and running in them. If you can feel an immediate, obvious relief in your feet and legs, then it's time to toss the old pair. In fact, some runners intentionally alternate between new and old shoes from day to day. This way, they retain their perception of what a fresh pair of shoes should feel like and are more likely to notice when the older pair is worn out.

Visible wear and tear. If the outsole is worn down to the midsole or the midsole is puckered and compressed, it means the shoes are clearly past their prime.

The shoe pitches. Shoes that no longer stand straight up and down have lost their structural integrity and are not able to protect you in the proper manner. Whether they pitch to the inside or the outside, it's time for them to go.

THE DO'S AND DON'TS OF SHOE CARE

DO . . .

• Keep shoes free of dirt with gentle hand washing.
• Dry shoes by loosening the laces, spreading the upper, removing the inner sock liner, and letting the shoe air-dry. Very wet shoes can be stuffed with newspaper, which will help to absorb moisture.
• Store shoes in a cool, dry environment. A hot car or humid garage will hasten the shoe's breakdown.

DON'T . . .

• Wash shoes in a washing machine.
• Dry shoes in a clothes dryer.
• Leave shoes to dry in direct sunlight. Strong sun can damage, dry, and shrink materials, making them more brittle and less effective over time.

THE LITTLE THINGS THAT COUNT

It's not just having the right running shoe that counts. How you wear your shoes and take care of your feet otherwise is also important. The following details can help keep you healthy and running comfortably.

Alternate between shoes. Take a tip from the pros and tailor your shoes to different workouts. Consider getting a pair of trail shoes for your trail runs, a beefier pair of shoes for your easy runs when speed is not important and comfort is key, and a lighter pair of shoes for racing and faster training days such as tempo runs and track workouts. Competitive runners are notorious for having a closet, even a garage, full of running shoes. While you don't need to go that far, alternating between two or three pairs is a good idea for any devoted runner.

Switching shoes on a regular basis accomplishes a few things. First, you allow your shoes to "recover" between uses, which means the midsole will not compress and deteriorate as rapidly. Second, you don't exacerbate minor pressure points that might be developing with any one particular pair of shoes. Third, in each different pair of shoes, your foot will land in a slightly different way, thus minimizing one of the causes of overuse injury—repeating the exact same motion over and over again. Even the slight change in foot placement you'll experience in a different pair of shoes is enough to rest your feet somewhat.

Don't wear new shoes on race day. New runners and racers typically make this mistake with the best of intentions. They think: "I want the best of all circumstances for my race, so I'll get some brand-new shoes."

The problem is that when you wear new shoes in a race situation, you haven't had a chance to test the shoes to determine if they are comfortable and appropriate for the speed and distance you'll be running. If they are not comfortable and you're in the middle of a race, chances are you'll continue to run in your less-than-optimal footwear. If you were just running a workout, you'd be more likely to stop and walk, intelligently cutting your losses.

In the span of a short race, blisters and pressure spots can easily develop in new shoes. In longer races, more serious issues also can arise if the shoe lacks adequate cushioning or motion control—one long race in the wrong shoes can actually mean the start of an injury.

Visit a running store. You get more knowledgeable service and a better selection of shoes, meaning you're more likely to find the best shoe for your needs.

Educate yourself about your foot type. The more you understand your foot, body, and stride type, the better you'll be able to determine if you're in appropriate shoes. This chapter provides a good overview to start with.

Invest in yourself. Be willing to buy good-quality shoes; remember, they're the only equipment you really need. Replace your shoes when they're worn out. Eking out extra miles on worn-out shoes can lead to injury.

What you really want for your race is "almost-new" shoes. Buy the shoes you wish to wear on race day several weeks ahead of time. First wear them on a few training runs of easy distance and then wear them at least once or twice for a faster workout such as a tempo run that will approximate race conditions. Use these runs to figure out if the shoes are comfortable and what socks you'll prefer to wear with them on race day.

Consider buying different shoes. Don't blindly buy the same model year after year. This might work for a while, but over time, the same shoe might not work so well for you. For one thing, manufacturers typically make changes to shoes each year—sometimes subtle, sometimes more radical. Beyond that, your own needs change with time. With age or weight gain, you might require a shoe with greater cushioning or more stability. After recuperating from an injury, you might find you have different requirements from a shoe.

If your old favorite doesn't feel as good as it used to, try on some different models from your favorite manufacturer or even experiment by revisiting some brands you'd sworn off—there's a chance that they've changed.

Wear comfortable street shoes. Since street shoes are what we wear most of the day, they are almost as important to a runner as running shoes. Granted, everyday shoes are not subjected to the same stresses and impact of running, but because we spend so many hours in them, they can exacerbate foot problems. Women especially are guilty of wearing flimsy footwear with no support and little cushioning.

When choosing your everyday shoes, look for adequate arch support and cushioning. Women should make sure the toe box has plenty of room, so that it is not squeezing the front of the foot into a pinched position. High heels are fine now and then, but avoid them on a daily basis, if possible. High heels shorten the Achilles tendon and place tremendous stress on the forefoot. These days, healthy, comfortable, and, yes, stylish alternatives exist, with slightly lower heels and better cushioning.

4

STRETCHING

INVESTING IN YOUR BODY

Here's what stretching can do for you.

- Increase your range of motion, which improves performance and makes running more comfortable

- Allow for optimal muscle function and stride length

- Provide a relaxing transition at the end of your run

- Help overworked muscles feel better

Here's what stretching can't do for you.

- Guarantee you a lifetime of injury-free running

It's true. Despite all the admonitions from experts to stretch, research never has proved beyond a doubt that stretching reduces the incidence of injury among runners. Most people are quick to blame injuries on not following a stretching program, says Tim Hilden, a physical therapist and gait analyst at the Boulder Center for Sports Medicine in Colorado. But nowadays we know that stretching isn't a panacea for all of a runner's ills. The fact remains that the primary causes of injury are (as discussed in the first chapters of this book) inappropriate training and a runner's individual biomechanics.

THE DO'S AND DON'TS OF STRETCHING

Stretching should not be considered a warm-up. It is much more effective as part of your cooldown routine.

DO . . .

Warm up beforehand. A "cold" muscle is more likely to strain than a warm one. On regular distance runs, jog slowly for several minutes before doing a few gentle stretches, then head into the bulk of your run. For races and track workouts, jog a few miles slowly first, then stretch, then run the workout. After the hard portion of the workout, another few slow miles can serve as a cooldown, which should be followed by a few minutes of stretching. Save the comprehensive stretch routine for after the run.

Stretch to your point of comfort. Overstretching can strain a muscle. Reach to a point of comfortable tension and then hold that position. Your range of motion eventually will improve.

Hold the stretch in a static position. Static stretching is safe as long as you are not reaching to the point of pain. When you are comfortable holding a position for 20 seconds, you can gradually increase the duration to 30 to 60 seconds.

DON'T . . .

Bounce. "Ballistic" stretching, as this is called, can contribute to muscle strains.

Stretch an injured muscle. If you're suffering from an injury, stretching can aggravate the area and prolong healing. Carefully stretch the surrounding and opposing muscles, but do not engage in any exercise that tugs on the damaged area.

Is that a reason not to spend time improving your flexibility? Not at all. Stretching *can* help prevent injury in certain cases. "Especially in individuals who are less flexible by nature," Hilden says. And it can be particularly effective in preventing a *recurrence* of injury, once potential trouble spots have made themselves known.

Besides, anecdotal evidence points strongly to the virtues of stretching. If you put enough miles on your legs, you can feel the difference when you stop stretching altogether. Range of motion is slowly reduced. Exercise can feel strained. Eventually, knotty, tender sections can develop in the workhorse muscles, such as the hamstrings, calf, and buttocks. When your body is that rigid and inflexible, you simply can't be running at optimal capacity. So a stretching routine remains a sensible part of a complete exercise program.

A REALISTIC APPROACH TO STRETCHING

You don't need to spend an hour a day grunting through a rigorous flexibility program. After all, most of us are busy enough trying to squeeze in our runs. Hilden, who has worked with runners of all abilities and ages on flexibility, strength, and biomechanics, knows that the average runner spends just a few minutes stretching. In fact, many runners don't take the time to stretch at all, thinking that flexibility is an all-or-nothing proposition—if they can't commit to half an hour a day, they do nothing at all.

With that in mind, Hilden developed two stretching programs specifically for this book. One consists of only the bare essentials and takes about 5 minutes—a "no excuses" routine that anyone can find time for. This program is designed to maximize the benefit of those few minutes of stretching, focusing on the areas of your body in which tightness is most likely to inhibit your running stride.

The second program is more comprehensive and tops out at about 20 to 25 minutes. This program has you holding each stretch for three repetitions instead of two. It also targets additional muscles that running tends to tighten in the hips, buttocks, and trunk.

THE QUICK PROGRAM

- *4 stretches*
- *Total time = 7 minutes*
- *Hold each stretch for 2 repetitions of 20 seconds on each side*

UPPER AND LOWER CALF

This stretch is particularly important for runners who suffer from plantar fasciitis.

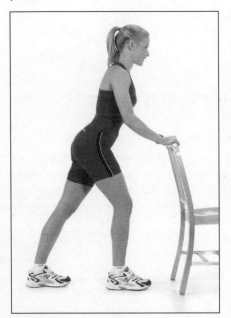 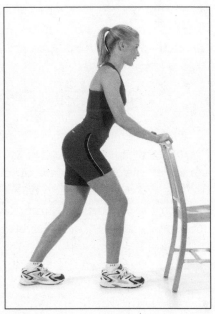

Start: Stand facing the back of a chair and place both hands on the chair for support. Take a step back with your left leg and extend it straight. Gently lean toward the chair so that you feel the stretch in your left calf. Don't let your ankle collapse; if your left foot falls inward, you won't stretch your calf properly. **Finish:** Bend the left leg at the knee. You should feel the stretch in your lower left calf.

HAMSTRING

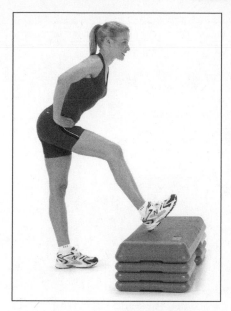 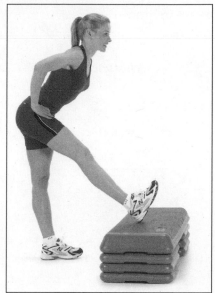

Start: Rest your right heel on a surface at least a foot off the floor but lower than hip level. (If your foot is too high, you'll stretch your back instead of your hamstring.) Bend your knee slightly. **Finish:** Slowly straighten the leg while leaning down slightly toward it. Keep your back straight and stable in order to keep the stretch in the hamstring area.

QUADRICEPS

Start: Stand straight, resting your left arm on a chair for balance. **Finish:** Bend your right knee, then grab your foot and pull it up toward your buttocks until you feel a comfortable stretch. Do not arch your back or lean in any direction.

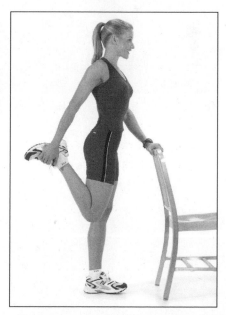

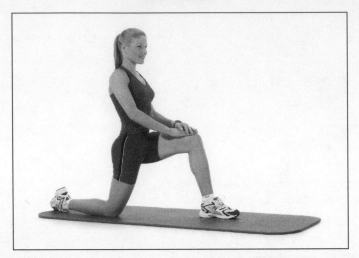

Start: Kneel on the floor and bring your left foot up onto the floor in front of you. (Place a towel or pad under your right knee if this is uncomfortable.) **Finish:** With your back straight, tuck and shift your pelvis slightly forward so that your right thigh is no longer perpendicular to the ground. You should feel the stretch in the front of the right leg.

THE COMPREHENSIVE PROGRAM

• *7 stretches (includes the Quick Program, plus the 3 additional stretches shown here)*

• *Total time = 20 minutes*

• *Hold each stretch for 3 repetitions of 20 to 30 seconds on each side*

ILIOTIBIAL BAND

The iliotibial (IT) band is a long stretch of connective tissue, and as such, it does not actually stretch. However, the areas where it attaches at the knee and hip are prime trouble spots for runners. Massaging the IT band with this exercise helps to loosen and work out kinks in the area.

Most gyms and health clubs now have rollers such as the one pictured here for stretching. You can also buy them at a sporting goods store. They are useful in stretching and massaging many other areas of the body.

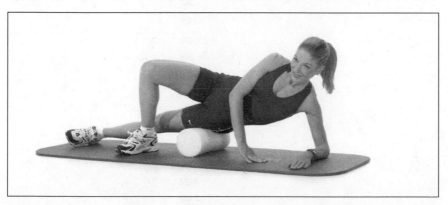

Start: Lie on your side, supporting your upper body with your arms. Place the roller under your left hip. **Finish:** With your back straight, roll up and down the entire length of the side of your thigh. Rest your right foot on the floor for balance or hold both feet off the floor. Start by slowly drawing your body across the roller, but if it feels good, you can move more briskly as well.

BUTTOCKS

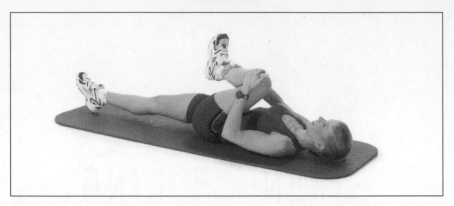

Lie on your back, bend your left knee, and lift your leg off the ground. Grasp your left ankle with your right hand and your left knee with your left hand. Gently pull your ankle to the right and push your knee toward your right shoulder until you feel a comfortable stretch.

TRUNK

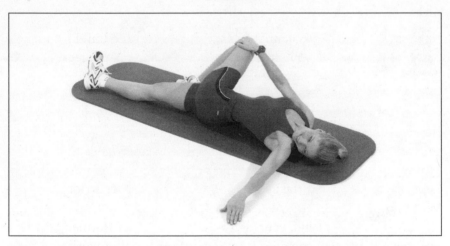

Lie on your back on the floor with your left arm straight out to the side and your head facing the left side. Bend your left knee up and across your body to the right. With your right hand, gently draw it toward the floor on your right side. Lock your left shoulder to the floor to keep as much of your back on the floor as possible.

5

STRENGTHENING

THE ICING ON THE CAKE

Running strengthens your legs but admittedly does little in the way of developing your upper body or midsection. Is that a problem? Should you spend time building muscle mass in your arms, trunk, or, for that matter, legs?

The answer depends on your goals and desires. If your goal is optimal racing and performance, building bulk is neither necessary nor desirable. In fact, competitive runners don't spend long hours in the weight room of the gym. Running requires—and tends to form—lean musculature that's better suited to endurance than power. However, some minimal strength work to supplement notable weak spots can help balance the body, generate power in your stride, and prevent injury.

If, on the other hand, your goal is to develop a well-formed physique and overall fitness, consider supplementing running workouts with strengthening exercises. You'll achieve a more balanced body, well-suited to all types of fitness endeavors, not to mention the physical stresses and requirements of ordinary life. As our bodies age, for example, a bad back or weak arms become more noticeable because they prevent us from carrying out everyday tasks—and running alone won't strengthen those areas.

Both of these goals are admirable, but another worthy goal is injury prevention. It's not as glamorous as winning races, but if you look at the body from a healthy-running perspective, the muscles of the core—your abdomen and back—take on significant importance. The muscles in the trunk area provide critical support for the mechanics of healthy running, and the best way to make sure they live up to that responsibility is to strengthen them.

Here's a look at the importance of supplementing with strength training, breaking the body down into its major components.

Upper body. For both running performance and injury prevention, building the upper body sits lowest on the priority list. For the most part, your arms are along for the ride in distance running. "You must have a minimum level of strength and endurance," says Neal Henderson, exercise physiologist and coordinator of sports science at the Boulder Center for Sports Medicine in Colorado. "But running tends to reduce muscle mass in the upper body, which is not necessarily a bad thing for performance." Simply put, the smaller the runner is on top, the less weight there is to haul around.

So strengthening your arms is largely a matter of personal preference. Some runners build arm strength for overall fitness, athletic ability, or even just aesthetics. Running does provide a bit of a head start: It burns calories and engages the arms secondarily, helping to define the muscles and improve arm endurance.

Trunk (abdomen and back). Unlike your arm muscles, which are not critical to running gait, your trunk (or core) is tremendously important to both running performance and injury prevention. And running doesn't do a whole lot to develop these areas. "You engage your core when you're running, but running itself doesn't provide a significant strengthening stimulus," says Tim Hilden, a physical therapist and gait analyst at the Boulder Center for Sports Medicine in Colorado.

"The core helps counteract the forces and stresses of running on the legs," says Henderson. If you don't strengthen your core, he warns, your form can deteriorate, leading to injuries. "Your upper body can twist and torque or collapse forward," he says. "Problems can start in your back and go all the way down through your legs."

Perhaps more than any other area of the body, core strength is integral to overall health and functioning (outside of the world of running), especially as we age. Maintaining a strong core can help fend off back

PERSONALIZING YOUR PROGRAM

The workouts described in this chapter are designed to fit the needs of runners in general. But many athletes might benefit from taking their strength program a step further and adding a few personalized exercises. If you're rehabbing from injury, for example, or if you have obvious biomechanical challenges, have your gait and musculature analyzed by a sports physician, trainer, or physical therapist who can then prescribe specific corrective exercises.

trouble, retain comfortable range of motion, and provide a foundation for other exercises and activities.

Legs. Obviously, running develops the legs. So there's some debate as to whether additional strength work is necessary for dedicated runners, especially among competitive runners. In one camp are athletes who feel that the legs—containing the workhorse muscles required for running—can never be strong enough. They often use weight machines or resistance bands in an effort to build overall strength, particularly during the winter or noncompetitive season.

In the other camp are runners who believe in specificity: meaning the act of running is the best training for running. Additional strength work, they feel, will only add bulk where it is not desirable. In addition, they fear that supplemental training needlessly tires the legs, resulting in poorer quality workouts on the track and roads, where it really counts.

Hilden recommends a middle ground. If you want to supplement your running with leg-strengthening exercises, be judicious about which muscles you work. For example, "you don't have to do a lot of calf raises," says Hilden. In fact, conventional leg-strengthening exercises performed on weight machines largely miss the point, he adds. Instead, it's the muscle groups nearby—those high up on the legs, closer to the trunk—that are important for both running performance and injury prevention. The hips and the glutes help move you forward. They also stabilize the leg and minimize torque, helping to prevent overuse injuries.

OPTIMIZING YOUR STRENGTHENING PROGRAM

Put it all together and it becomes clear that a runner's optimal strength program for both performance and injury prevention should target the midsection of the body as if it were a bull's-eye. Your time and effort are best spent developing the core muscles, after which you should focus on the "circle" beyond the trunk—the upper back, hips, and buttocks. Low on the priority list are the extremities—the lower legs and arms.

Hilden devised the following strength program solely for this book. It's designed primarily to reduce your likelihood of injury and secondarily to enhance running performance.

It was also designed with reality in mind. Most runners don't have an hour a day to spend on a strength workout, so we created two workout options. The Quick Program boils down strengthening for runners to the bare essentials. When you're short on time or motivation, you can do these exercises a few times a week in just minutes a day. Hilden says he can't guarantee you'll remain injury-free, but you'll place yourself miles ahead of other runners who don't do any supplemental strength work. The Comprehensive Program builds on the Quick Program, adding several additional exercises to target more of the body. If and when you have the time, this workout is advisable.

Feel free to combine programs to fit your schedule. For example, you can do the Quick Program on most days and try to add the Comprehen-

HOW TO CHOOSE DUMBBELLS

The best way to work the biceps is with actual weights. If you don't have access to dumbbells at a gym, buy some at a sporting goods store. They are inexpensive and versatile, lending themselves to many other upper-body exercises, including those for the triceps and shoulder muscles.

When buying dumbbells, choose a weight with which you can just barely complete your 10 required repetitions. Buy that set and the next heavier weight. When you can easily complete 15 repetitions with the lighter weight, move up to the next set.

sive Program twice a week when your schedule allows. As your body gets stronger, each program gets harder. When you can perform the exercises without feeling muscle fatigue, look for the words "When You Get Good" and follow those directions.

THE QUICK PROGRAM

- *3 exercises*
- *Total time = 10 minutes*

BALANCE BALL CURLS

This all-in-one exercise utilizes many of the core muscles as well as those of the gluteus. It's an intense hamstring strengthener as well. It looks like play but provides a whopper of a workout.

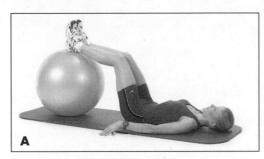

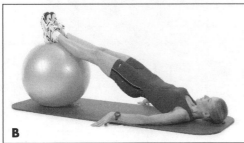

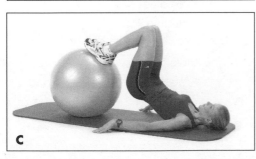

Lie on the floor, bend your knees almost 90 degrees, and rest your heels on top of the exercise ball (A). With your arms resting on the floor for support and your abdominal muscles holding your trunk and pelvis still, lift your buttocks and lower back off the floor, so that you're resting on your shoulders and upper back. Then extend your legs fully so they form a straight line with your body (B). Bend your knees and curl your legs inward as far as possible, rotating the ball toward your body with your feet (C).

When you get good: When you get good at balance ball curls, try this variation. Instead of placing both legs on the ball, rest just your right leg on it. Keep your left leg stationary and straight just above the ball. Using your abdominal muscles to hold your trunk and pelvis still, extend your right leg fully. Bend your right knee and curl your legs inward as far as possible, rotating the ball toward you with your feet. Do 3 sets of 10 with each leg.

SKATING SWINGS

Many running injuries stem from a repeated collapsing action of the knee, which leads to excessive internal rotation of the femur (thigh bone) and over-pronation. That motion can also result from weaknesses higher up in the leg. Strengthening the hip and gluteus (buttocks) muscles helps keep the entire leg aligned. If you don't have access to a gym, you can do the next two exercises at home using resistance tubing or stretch bands (available at most sporting goods stores). Anchor the tubing low to the ground, around a couch or table leg, for example. If you do these exercises with cables at the gym, choose a weight that provides some resistance but not so much that you can't maintain proper form. If you must arch and sway your back in order to swing your leg, the resistance is too heavy.

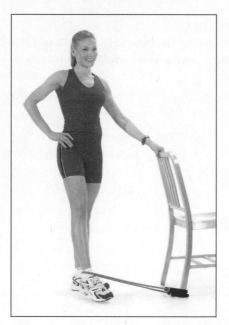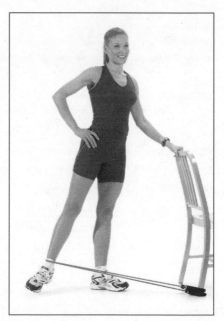

Start: Loop a resistance band or exercise cable around your right foot. Face the point of resistance and step back until the band is taut. Then rotate your body about 45 degrees to the right. Keep your pelvis squared in this direction and your back straight. Relax your right leg and let the band pull it toward the point of resistance with your toe pointing forward. **Finish.** Keeping your right leg straight, extend it back. As you pull your leg back, rotate the foot outward as much as you can. Don't arch your back or "rock" in order to extend the leg. Do 3 sets of 10 with each leg. **When you get good:** Increase to 4 sets.

SOCCER KICKS

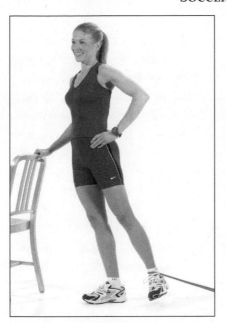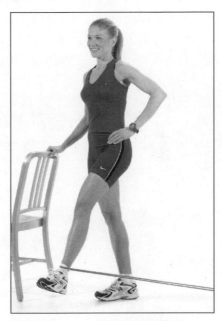

Start: Loop a resistance band or exercise cable around your left foot and face away from the point of resistance. Rest your right hand on a sturdy object for support. Step forward until the band is taut. Then rotate your body about 45 degrees to the left. Keeping your pelvis still, relax your left leg and let the band pull it back toward the point of resistance. **Finish:** Swing your left leg forward (keeping it straight) with your foot rotated slightly outward, as if you were kicking a soccer ball. Do 3 sets of 10 repetitions with each leg. **When you get good:** Increase to 4 sets.

THE COMPREHENSIVE PROGRAM

• *9 exercises (includes the Quick Program, plus the following 6 additional exercises)*

• *Total time = 45 minutes*

SUPINE BRIDGES

This exercise targets a number of critical areas, including the core stability muscles, gluteus, and hip flexors.

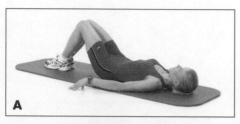

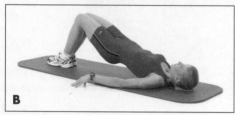

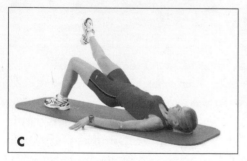

Lie faceup on the floor with your knees bent and your pelvis tucked under to keep the small of your back flat on the floor (A). With your arms resting on the floor for support, raise your hips and buttocks off the floor, creating a straight line from your shoulders to your knees (B). Lift your right leg off the floor and extend it straight out. Then extend it out to the side as far as comfortable (C). Return your leg to the center position and lower it. Do 3 sets of 10 repetitions on each side. **When you get good:** Increase to 3 sets of 15 repetitions.

LEG EXTENSIONS

This movement utilizes the lower abdominal muscles, an area in which runners are notoriously underdeveloped. It also targets other core stabilizing muscles.

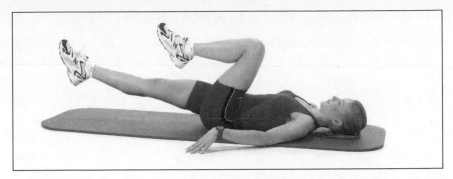

Start: Lie faceup on the floor with your pelvis tucked under slightly and your abdominals contracted to keep your back flat on the floor. With your arms resting on the floor for support, lift both legs off the floor so your knees are in line with your hips. **Finish:** Extend your right leg while pulling your left leg back, then extend your left leg while pulling your right leg back (that's 1 repetition). Do 3 sets of 10 repetitions. **When you get good:** Increase to 3 sets of 15 repetitions.

WALL SQUATS

This exercise looks simple but provides a wicked workout. These squats primarily target the quadriceps. To work the gluteus muscles to a greater degree, tighten them during the exercise.

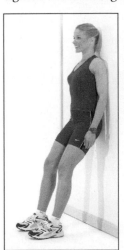
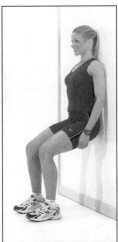

Start: Stand back against a wall with your pelvis tucked under slightly to keep your entire back touching the wall. Walk your feet out from the wall about a foot and a half, keeping them roughly shoulder-width apart. **Finish:** Keeping your back on the wall, bend your legs and slide into a squatting position. Make sure your knees do not go out farther than your toes, since this will place excess strain on the knees. Straighten the legs to return to the starting position. Do 4 sets of 10 repetitions. **When you get good:** Hold your body in the squatting position for an extra 5, 10, even 30 seconds at several points throughout the workout.

BICEPS CURLS

Since running itself does little to develop the arms, a few arm and shoulder exercises are not a bad idea. Plus, strengthening the shoulders contributes to better posture, which in turn can prevent injury.

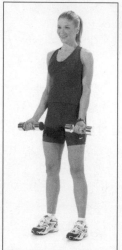 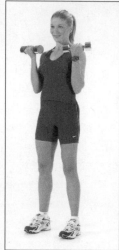

Start: Grab a dumbbell in each hand. Stand with your arms down at your sides and your back straight. Keep your legs straight without locking your knees. **Finish:** With your palms facing up, raise the dumbbells toward your shoulders. Then lower your arms slowly—momentum won't help you get strong. Do 3 sets of 10 repetitions. **When you get good:** Do 4 sets or increase your weight slightly.

TRICEPS EXTENSIONS

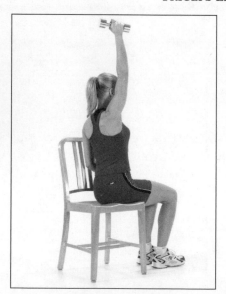 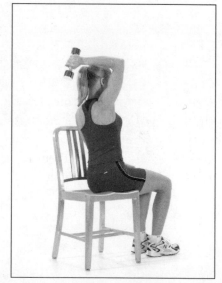

Start: Sit sideways on a chair or weight bench. Grab a dumbbell with your right hand and raise it straight up over your head, palm facing inward toward your head. **Finish:** Slowly lower the weight at an angle behind your head toward your left ear, keeping your arm close to your head. Repeat. Do 3 sets of 10 repetitions with each arm. When you get good: Increase to 4 sets.

SHOULDER ABDUCTIONS

This exercise works the shoulders, arms, and back. Anchor resistance tubing around a solid object near your waist level.

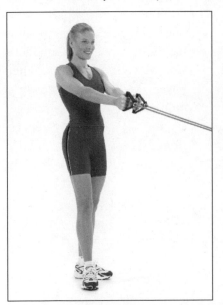 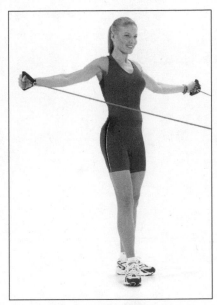

Start: Grab each end of a resistance tube and stand facing the point of resistance with your arms straight out in front of you. Step back until the tube is taut, then step forward with one leg for balance. **Finish:** Keeping your back and arms straight, slowly bring both arms out to each side. Then slowly bring them back to the starting position. Do 3 sets of 10 repetitions. **When you get good:** Increase to 4 sets.

6

CROSS-TRAINING

THE RUNNER'S INSURANCE POLICY

Most runners love the simplicity of running. Step after step, step after step—it's a meditation of movement. If we didn't love the very action of putting one foot in front of the other endlessly, we'd never have become runners. But with every footfall, we inflict the same, repetitive stress on our bodies. And you know now that those repetitive stresses can result in injury.

Earlier in this book, I covered some of the ways you can avoid injury, from training correctly to choosing proper shoes. Now I'm going to address a way in which you can avoid some of the repetition altogether: by cross-training.

Cross-training is just another way of saying variety. The term has taken on a technical tone that intimidates some runners and exercisers, but in practice cross-training doesn't have to be scientific or complicated. The general idea is to go out and have some fun doing things that give your body a break from running.

Cross-training can mean anything from taking a walk to going skiing. For some people, a relaxing weekly yoga class is the extent of their cross-training. For others, a more formal cross-training regimen might include a combination of strength training, swimming, and cycling. Take whatever approach appeals to you and helps you meet your goals.

THE BENEFITS OF CROSS-TRAINING

The principle behind cross-training is that by engaging in activities that complement your primary sport, you can make fitness gains that do not stress your body in the same way. This reduces your risk of injury and enhances your performance. It holds true for all sports but is particularly helpful in running because of its repetitive nature. Cross-training helps runners in a variety of ways. It develops muscular and cardiovascular fitness in a comprehensive manner, it lowers risk of injury, and it maintains fitness during injury rehabilitation.

"Any runner can benefit from cross-training," says Neal Henderson, exercise physiologist and coordinator of sports science at the Boulder Center for Sports Medicine in Colorado. But injury-prone runners in particular have the most to gain. These runners have problems simply because their bodies cannot tolerate a high volume of training, probably due to anatomical inefficiencies. They tend to get injured repeatedly, despite their best efforts to train intelligently. "Cross-training allows these runners to develop aerobic fitness and muscular endurance using other activities," Henderson says.

Other runners benefit for similar reasons.

New runners. Experts say other types of exercise should be virtually mandatory for beginners. That's because novice runners have bodies that are not conditioned to the stresses of running. They should be running only every other day or, at most, 2 days in a row. So supplementing with another sport or activity until the body can handle more running is an excellent strategy for getting in shape.

Recreationally competitive runners. Experienced runners still benefit from cross-training. There's only so much running you can do, Henderson explains. Yet total training volume—meaning all varieties of exercise a runner engages in—has a direct impact on performance. So to boost performance without adding risk of injury, the answer for runners who are already doing high mileage is to supplement their running with something else. "Serious runners are close to their upper limit of running, but with cross-training, they can get that little bit more without risking injury," Henderson says. Cross-training can help these runners mentally as well. Some runners become stale and uninspired when they're doing heavy training; a variety of sports can keep things feeling fresh.

Older runners. As we age, our bodies become less flexible. We also

THE LIMITS OF CROSS-TRAINING

If cross-training is so great, why don't professional runners do more of it? Because to become a faster runner, one must run—fast. As overall fitness increases, only one-sport training will make athletes better at their designated sport.

Cross-training for top-caliber runners can be more detrimental than helpful for a few reasons. First, professional runners train at the limits of endurance. They run very high mileage, much of it at a very high intensity. That means they must conserve all their energy for their running workouts. They're already as fit as they can be, so biking or hiking won't make them run faster; these sports will just make them better bikers or hikers.

Second, these runners are far more efficient than the average runner. Professional runners train twice or even three times a day. If they had significant anatomical challenges that made them injury-prone, they'd never survive the rigors of their training. So using cross-training to take a break from the stresses of running becomes less important. They are less likely to get hurt than you or I.

The cross-training that elite runners do tends to focus on stretching, since running has a tightening effect on the body. These activities don't build fitness so much as they relax and loosen the body. Favorite choices include swimming, yoga, and Pilates.

Finally, some pros also enjoy other activities when they're taking their break from training. Over the winter, for example, they might take up skiing or cycling for a change. But when they return to training, chances are they'll become one-sport wonders again.

What does it mean to you? Unless you're an elite runner, you probably still can benefit from cross-training. But the more serious a runner you are, the more specificity of training will benefit you, too.

If you're a serious competitor, limit your cross-training to a few times a week. Engage in activities that you can do in *addition* to running (not instead of) and that loosen your muscles. And save the biking, skiing, or rock climbing for the off-season, when you're not racing.

lose muscle mass and strength. Both of these tendencies can make runners more prone to injury. By engaging in cross-training, older runners can maintain fitness without running every day. Specifically, activities that don't pound the joints, such as swimming, cycling, or cross-country skiing, are excellent for the aging runner.

COMBINING RUNNING WITH OTHER ACTIVITIES

Newer runners and runners who are predisposed to injury can devote 50 percent of their overall workout time to cross-training. You might do this by running every other day and doing other activities on the off days.

Some days you can combine workouts, running for a shorter period of time and then doing something else: a swim at the pool or a spinning class at the gym. It's crucial to take days off from running, however—if you cut your run time in half and still do it every day, you're not reaping the full benefit of cross-training.

Choose activities you enjoy and let your imagination run wild. Even a game of Frisbee can be considered cross-training if it's played with

WHAT YOU CAN DO

CROSS-TRAINING FOR BEGINNING RUNNERS

New runners can incorporate cross-training into their schedules as a way to prevent injury early in a running program. Here's a sample schedule of what a typical week might look like. Of course, you can vary the activities based on what you enjoy and have access to.

Monday—jog 30 minutes
Tuesday—swim 45 minutes
Wednesday—jog 30 minutes
Thursday—rest day or hike
Friday—exercise bike or yoga class
Saturday—jog 45 minutes
Sunday—rest day or jog 30 minutes

CROSS-TRAINING FOR EXPERIENCED RUNNERS

Experienced and competitive runners can handle more training. Cross-training serves to alleviate the pounding at least once a week and supplements fitness. Here's a sample schedule.

Monday—run 45 minutes
Tuesday—track workout
Wednesday—run 45 to 60 minutes
Thursday—swim 45 minutes
Friday—tempo run
Saturday—jog 30 minutes easy; Pilates class
Sunday—long run of 90 minutes

enough vigor to get your heart rate up. Don't do a sport because you feel you must—if cross-training feels like drudgery, you won't stick with it and won't reap the benefits.

When possible, complement running with non-weight-bearing activities that give your legs a complete break from pounding. Swimming and cycling are the classic cross-training choices for runners because they are gentler on your joints.

As you become more experienced with and serious about your running, the focus of your cross-training should change. Instead of splitting your time between running and other activities, shift the balance. Running should take up the majority of your training time, with cross-training as a supplement just once or twice a week.

Use cross-training as a way to get some conditioning work done on rest days from running. This way, you're resting your legs from the pounding but still building fitness. Or do it after a run as a way to build strength in other areas of the body or to enhance flexibility.

More serious runners also should be choosier about their cross-training activities. If you are racing, in particular, choose sports and exercise that enhance, rather than detract from, your running. That means activities that lengthen and loosen muscles (such as swimming, yoga, and Pilates), rather than tighten them (like weight training or cycling).

CROSS-TRAINING ACTIVITIES

Here's a look at some of the most popular cross-training activities and how they can be incorporated into your running.

Water Running

Best for: impact-related injuries, such as plantar fasciitis or stress fractures.

What it's all about. Water running is the sole purview of die-hard runners. It is just what it sounds like: running in the water. Not very exciting, to be sure. But if you're an injured—and frustrated—runner, then water running can be just what the doctor ordered.

Water running allows an athlete to very closely approximate the motion of his or her favorite sport, reaping many of the benefits of running with no impact whatsoever. Serious runners who don't want to lose their hard-won fitness gains while injured will find water running to be a terrific cross-training option. Water running works because your body goes through the same motions as during a run, utilizing many of the same muscles and boosting your heart rate. In fact, it's a double whammy, since the added resistance of water makes it a more intense strength workout than regular running. Because of the increased resistance against your legs, water running can aggravate some injuries, including muscle strains. So use caution when running in the water, and listen to your body.

Some (very dedicated) runners incorporate water running into their training when they are not injured. They hope that by substituting 1 day of training per week with a water run, they'll give their legs a break from the pounding of the roads and buy an insurance policy against injury. It certainly couldn't hurt, although most runners will find it's just too tedious to do unless they are injured.

Studies have shown that injured runners who train in the water rigorously while rehabbing find that they are able to maintain a great degree of fitness. If you rehab in this manner, be careful when you return to the roads. Your heart, lungs, and muscles might be raring to go, but your joints and connective tissue will have deconditioned. You'll still need to return gradually to your regular training. Resume by alternating days in the pool with days of running on a soft surface such as grass or wood chips.

Unlike most other cross-training activities, water running is something you probably haven't done before. Here's some basic instruction to get you started.

To run in the water, you'll need a special flotation device designed just for this purpose. These are available at large sporting goods stores and running stores, and some pools will have them available for you to borrow.

Strap on your flotation vest and head to the deep end of the pool. Make sure it's deep enough that your feet don't touch the ground. Start to run, using the same posture and stride you would on the ground. If you are doing this correctly, you will barely move forward in the water.

The biggest mistake runners make in the water is that they think they must cover ground quickly, so they invariably hunch forward, bending at the waist. By doing so, you will move forward more, but you'll basically be doggie-paddling. This is not an effective workout, and you're not getting the benefits you would be from running.

You'll quickly notice that water running is dull. After 10 minutes, you'll probably feel like you've been in the pool for half an hour. To make things more interesting—and to get a better workout—try approximating your usual running workouts by varying your intensity. Any workout you can do on a road or track you can do in the water (with the exception of hills, obviously). You vary your intensity by pumping faster, although you won't actually move forward that much in the water.

For example, do an interval workout like this: Warm up by jogging slowly in the water for 10 minutes. Then run hard in the water for 1 minute. Remember, don't lean over—the goal is not to cover more ground—just retain your good running posture and pump your arms and legs faster. (You might be amazed at how challenging this is. Don't go too fast or you'll tire before the minute is up.) After 1 minute of "running fast," water jog slowly for a minute to recover. Repeat this process for as long as you want.

Ladders are another good water workout: Run hard for 1 minute, then jog slowly, then run hard for 2 minutes, then 3, and so on, always jogging slowly between. You'll soon get a sense of pacing, just as you would on the track, and see how hard you can push for each length of time.

Swimming

Best for: rehabilitation from most injuries, fitness training for new runners, fitness supplementation for veteran runners.

(continued on page 76)

PERSONAL TRAINERS VERSUS RUNNING COACHES

Personal trainers are increasingly popular with people who simply want to get in shape. They create training schedules, supervise workouts, and provide motivation. Trainers are often proponents of cross-training, since doing a variety of activities is a good idea for newcomers to fitness and for people who are attempting to lose weight. Many people who enjoy working with a trainer say they are more likely to stick with their program because of the one-on-one interaction.

That's all good. And if you're just beginning a running program, working with a trainer is not a bad idea. But as you become more experienced and more serious about the sport, the benefits of a trainer decrease. That's because a general trainer will make you generally fit; if you want to be fit specifically for running, you need to follow a program designed specifically for running. And most personal trainers don't know a whole lot about running per se—they focus their attention instead on sports and activities that you can do in a gym.

If you're getting serious about running, consider swapping your personal trainer for a running coach. Or join a local running club. You still can incorporate cross-training into your workout plan, but you'll do so with an eye toward your overall running.

Whichever your preference, here's how to find someone you can work with.

Ask around. If you belong to a health club, begin your search for a trainer there. If you don't belong to a club, ask around for word-of-mouth recommendations.

To find a coach, visit your local running store and look for fliers or advertisements. Also ask the sales help if they know of local coaches. You can also call the area running club for names.

Look for like-mindedness. When interviewing trainers, look for compatible personalities. Some trainers have the style of a drill sergeant, others of a best friend offering motivation—choose a trainer with whom you'll feel comfortable. Ask about their experience and be sure that your own goals are something the trainer understands and has the knowledge to help you with.

When you're interviewing coaches, ask what type of runners they train. Some coaches specialize in training fast runners, while others work with beginners. Ask about the coach's training philosophy, whether you'll train with other runners, whether the coach goes to the workouts, and how often he'll give you a schedule or meet with you for feedback. Ideally, find a coach who trains other runners who have similar abilities and goals.

Many coaches now offer online services, e-mail schedules, and phone consultations. Because these coaches won't be able to see you run in person, they can't gauge how you feel on a particular day and see your fitness progress—they'll rely on your feedback for that. Also, they won't be on hand the day of a hard workout to provide motivation. For these reasons, online coaching is better for more experienced runners who know how to listen to their bodies and who don't mind not having a cheerleader on the sidelines.

Check out qualifications. Trainers can be certified by several different organizations, the most reputable being the American College of Sports Medicine (ACSM) and the American Council on Exercise. Look for a trainer with a degree in exercise science or a health-related field, such as kinesiology. The ACSM Web site can help you find a trainer in your area with its ProFinder feature; go to www.acsm.org. Ask for references and check certifications.

When choosing a coach, ask about his or her experience. Many will not be formally certified, having gained their experience from years of training themselves and other athletes.

Consider your budget. Trainers charge anywhere from $40 to $100 per hour.

Coaches' fees range from $50 to $150 a month, depending on how often they meet with you and how detailed their training information is.

What it's all about. Swimming is a wonderful complement to running, providing a relaxing, healthy break with no force of impact on your body. Swimming develops the arms and trunk, notoriously underutilized in running. It also tends to lengthen and stretch muscles, rather than tighten them.

Runners can swim through almost any injury. Because the entire stride and foot-strike biomechanics are removed from the equation, swimming is safe while you're rehabbing from most foot, ankle, knee, and hip injuries. For this same reason, you will lose some of your running-specific conditioning if you are solely on a swimming program, but you can maintain cardiovascular fitness and avoid weight gain.

For healthy runners, swimming provides a good counterpart to any training program. New runners can alternate running and swimming days, increasing their fitness without pounding their legs every day. Veteran runners should use swimming as a supplement to running, not instead of it. In fact, swimming is one of the few cross-training activities that professional runners engage in with regularity, since it provides a relaxing, nontightening workout—a fitness bonus for the day that doesn't detract from the serious work of running. You can easily swim on the same day as a run since it doesn't stress the same muscles and doesn't contribute any impact to the joints. Or you might swim on your 1 day a week off from running.

Cycling

Best for: maintaining fitness while rehabbing impact-related injuries, such as plantar fasciitis or stress fractures. Depending on the specifics, cycling might aggravate knee and ankle injuries, since these joints do move (albeit without impact) while you're cycling.

What it's all about. Cycling is a good aerobic and muscular workout. It works the leg muscles more intensely than running, particularly the medial quadriceps (the tops of your thighs) and calf muscles. That's a good counterpart to running, since running tends to build the hamstrings and lateral quads. Cycling is also an impact-free workout, another reason it's a good complement to running.

In order to reap comparable benefits from a bike ride, you'll have to ride for a longer duration than if you were running. (One rule of thumb is to double the length of time you'd be running to get the same workout benefits from a bike ride. So if you'd be running half an hour, ride for an hour.)

Cycling is a great activity for beginning runners who want to get in shape. It can complement their training on nonrunning days. Since new-comers to the sport shouldn't run every day, they can still burn calories and get an aerobic workout on a bike. While competitive runners typi-cally avoid the bike because it develops such different musculature in the legs, many older runners rediscover the activity when they cut back the number of days they run.

Use whatever type of bike you prefer; the fitness benefits are similar. Exercise and spinning bikes found in health clubs are fine, and some people like the option of watching television or reading a magazine (something you can't do while running). Getting outside on a real bike might provide more inspiration—and therefore a longer workout. Real bikes do have drawbacks though: They are expensive, and maintaining gear can be time-consuming.

Nordic (Cross-Country) Skiing

Best for: rehabbing most injuries where impact and foot strike are problematic; for example, coming back from a stress fracture or getting over plantar fasciitis or runner's knee.

What it's all about. Nordic skiing is quite possibly the best cross-training conditioner for runners. It provides overall conditioning, and you can substitute it for running during the winter. Like running, it of-fers great rewards for the heart and lungs. Cross-country skiing also builds leg strength but requires more from the trunk and upper body than running does, because of the arm motion involved. That means it's an even more comprehensive full-body workout than running. Finally, and best of all for runners, there's no impact. Runners can ski all day long and still give their joints a break.

Downhill skiing does less to condition the body than Nordic skiing. While it does give the quadriceps a good workout, it provides a relatively short duration of activity punctuated by rest (on the chairlift). Plus, gravity does most of the work pulling you downhill. It's better to think of downhill skiing as an occasional break rather than as a serious condi-tioning workout. Besides, many runners are wary of downhill skiing be-cause of the considerable possibility of twisting a knee in a fall. If you're training seriously and don't want to be sidelined by a nonrunning injury, you're better off sticking to cross-country skiing.

Snowshoeing

Best for: overall fitness. Because the motion so closely approximates running, this is not the best activity for rehabbing running injuries that involve the knee joint, Achilles tendon, or foot pain.

What it's all about. Snowshoeing has exploded in popularity and for good reason: It's easy, cheap, and fun, and there's virtually no learning curve involved. Buy or rent a pair of snowshoes, strap them on, and walk out into the snow. Within less than a minute, you'll feel comfortable enough to start jogging. That's it. There's no technique to learn, no equipment to master.

As with running, snowshoeing is a quick, efficient workout. If you live in a cold climate where you have access to trails and wilderness, buying a pair of snowshoes is a good fitness investment—they can get you outside when the roads are snowed under. Choose a narrow, light-weight pair designed for running, which will allow you to most closely approximate your natural running stride. (Wider, heavier snowshoes intended for backcountry excursions will force you to plant your feet farther apart than you're normally accustomed to.)

Since you can jog on snowshoes, this workout can give you benefits similar to a run. You won't be able to go as fast, but the added resistance on your feet means you'll be getting a bonus strength workout for your legs. Despite your slower pace, chances are your heart will be working just as hard, if not harder. And even though you're running, snowshoeing results in less impact to your legs because the snow provides a soft surface.

Pilates and Yoga

Best for: recovering from most injuries—just skip any positions that aggravate the injury site or cause pain, and clear the activity with your doctor first. You can do either on the same day as a run or on your day off from running.

What they're all about. Both these activities are beneficial regular supplements to your running program. There are many different types of yoga, but all focus to some degree on flexibility, strengthening, and breathing—all of which are complementary to the tightening effects of running. Pilates is an intense workout that imparts both strength and

A WORD ABOUT TEAM SPORTS

Kicking or tossing a ball around with a bunch of friends is a fun way to spend your time but doesn't necessarily offer reliable fitness benefits. Activities such as football and softball entail a lot of standing around—and not a lot of actual exercise. Sports that require more continuous movement, such as soccer and basketball, result in a better workout. The best rule of thumb when considering team sports as part of your cross-training is to play if you enjoy them, but do so in addition to your regular running or other workouts, not instead of them.

While you're playing, be sensible about your abilities and exertion level. Team sports generally require short, fast bursts of action. This is the opposite of what you're conditioned for as a runner. If you're overzealous while sprinting to catch a ball or trying to make it to first base, you could easily pay the price with a muscle or tendon strain.

---

flexibility. Neither of these activities is considered an aerobic workout (although you probably will break a sweat).

It's best to do both yoga and Pilates on a continuing, long-term basis. The learning curve is a bit steep: You'll definitely need instruction, and the longer you go to classes, the better and more comfortable you'll become at the required exercises.

Traditional Pilates requires a set of unique equipment and machines (which can be found at fitness clubs and dedicated Pilates studios), and lessons are not cheap. However, many instructors offer mat classes—sessions of exercises conducted solely on the floor without the special equipment—that are more affordable and provide a good introduction to the discipline.

I can't overstate the benefits of these disciplines for all runners. Pilates and yoga are both more effective at increasing range of motion than simple stretching. They strengthen the core and the smaller muscles throughout the body that are necessary for stabilization. All this helps your posture and stride as a runner and, in some cases, will keep injuries at bay.

7

FORCES OF NATURE

RUNNING HOT, RUNNING COLD

We runners love our sport because we can do it virtually anytime, anywhere. When baseball games are cancelled due to rain, we runners happily splash through the puddles. When tennis players and golfers store their equipment for the winter, we break out our high-tech jackets and tights. And when all the sane and sedentary folks retire indoors to watch an air-conditioned movie, we runners slog through the heat of summer, too.

There's little that Mother Nature can devise that will stop a runner intent on a daily workout. That's one of the beauties of running. But this die-hard attitude also can spell trouble. When the meteorologist admonishes folks to stay indoors or not to partake in strenuous activity because of a heat wave, most runners assume that's guidance for everybody else—not them.

It's true that if you are in good running shape, you are also probably better able to handle some challenging conditions and hardships. But that doesn't make you immune to the elements. Illnesses brought on by heat and cold, while not technically running injuries, are some of the more serious—and common—conditions that runners face. What follows is a look at safety precautions that are a good idea for all runners, regardless of fitness or ability.

RUNNING IN THE HEAT

The most serious problem resulting from running in hot weather is heat illness, which, thankfully, is easy to prevent. Unfortunately, it's also easy to ignore, which makes it surprisingly dangerous, especially for runners who think they are immune to the elements. A number of factors determine how susceptible you'll be to heat illness. Obesity, lack of fitness, a recent illness, sleep deprivation, and sunburn all increase your risk.

Because heat illness proceeds in three stages, each with its own warning signs, it's important to understand the symptoms.

Stage 1: Heat Cramps

What's happening. Muscles spasm painfully from dehydration and loss of electrolytes through sweat without proper replenishment of fluids. Essentially, your body is hoarding its liquids and precious blood supply for the essential organs and brain, compromising the muscles.

What to do. Stop running. Gradually sip liquids; some form of sports drink or juice is preferable to water. (When the body sweats, it doesn't lose just water but also electrolytes such as sodium and potassium. It's important to replace these minerals, too.) If no such drink is available, drink water, but also try to take in some salty snacks, such as pretzels or a sports bar. Stop your workout if possible and gently massage your muscles. If you must continue exerting yourself (to get back to your car or a trailhead), wait for the cramping to abate and then walk. If possible, continue to hydrate while you make your way back.

Heat cramps themselves are not dangerous, but they are a warning of more trouble to come. When an athlete (or anybody, for that matter) suffering from heat cramps ignores the symptoms and continues exertion, the illness can worsen rapidly to heat exhaustion and eventually heatstroke. Do not ignore cramping and do not attempt to finish your workout without addressing the problem.

Stage 2: Heat Exhaustion

What's happening. In a state of heat exhaustion, body temperature rises due to exertion and weather conditions, and sweating depletes the body's fluids. Blood volume decreases. Blood pressure drops, and with it, the following symptoms are possible: fainting, dizziness, weakness, a rapid and weak pulse, pale skin that feels clammy, prickly heat, goose

WHAT YOU CAN DO

Focus on avoiding heat illness and you should never have to worry about treating it. Follow these guidelines.

Avoid midday exertion. Exercise in the cooler hours of early morning and late evening.

Check the weather. When you do, be aware not just of the temperature but also of the heat index, a measurement that combines temperature with relative humidity. High humidity raises the risk of suffering heat illness, since the body's evaporative cooling system does not work as efficiently in moist conditions as it does in drier ones.

Stay out of the sun. Look for running routes shaded by trees.

Slow your pace. The higher your level of exertion, the more heat you generate and the harder your body has to work to cool itself.

Stay hydrated. Drink throughout the day and have a cup of water or sports drink within the half hour before your run. For runs of more than 1 hour, carry a sports drink to replace electrolytes lost in sweating. (For more specifics on fluids, see the section on hydration on page 84.)

Dress properly. Wear a lightweight running cap or sun visor to keep the sun off your face. Wear lightweight, wicking fabrics designed specifically for running in hot weather. These will facilitate your body's cooling process by allowing your sweat to evaporate.

Protect your skin. Use a water-resistant sunblock lotion, which can help keep the body cool by minimizing the sun's burning effects.

Get acclimated. If you've just traveled to a hot, humid climate, your body will be less able to handle the weather conditions. Avoid strenuous exertion for prolonged periods, instead building up gradually over the course of a week or so.

Listen to your body. Recognize and heed the early signs of heat illness (see above). Remember, while heat cramps and exhaustion are themselves not dangerous, they are the first steps on the way to heatstroke, a potentially fatal condition. Never ignore or "push through" heat cramps and exhaustion. Stop running immediately and get out of the sun. Rest and hydrate, hydrate, hydrate with a sports drink or water, along with a little food.

pimples, cramps, chills, nausea, vomiting, clumsiness, hyperventilating, and confusion.

What to do. Cease running immediately. Sit down and rest, and if possible, get out of the sun and into a cool spot. Drink a sports drink or water. Take small sips to avoid aggravating your system. (If you are unable to keep liquids down, get medical help—since hydrating is now essential.) If plenty of water or ice is available, also use it directly on your skin to cool it.

Stage 3: Heatstroke

What's happening. Heatstroke is the final stage of heat illness, and it is potentially fatal. Essentially, the body has lost its ability to regulate its temperature. Severe dehydration compromises the ability to sweat, which means core temperature rises to dangerous levels. Organ function is impaired, and left untreated, the condition can be fatal. Symptoms of heatstroke are hot, red, dry skin; rapid heart rate; disorientation; and eventually loss of consciousness.

What to do. Seek medical help. Heatstroke is a medical emergency and must be treated at once. Meanwhile, the body should be cooled immediately, by any means available. Use water or ice packs on the skin and move the victim out of the sun.

THE (NEW) HYDRATION EQUATION

For many years, experts have strongly advised runners to drink early and often during workouts and races. Drink before you get thirsty, we've been told. Drink as much as you can on the run. And finish every run with another big bottle of water.

The strict warnings have come because sweat evaporation is the primary method by which your body cools itself. Without enough fluid available—in other words, when you're dehydrated—your ability to sweat is compromised. Not enough fluids equals not enough sweat. And without enough sweat, your body begins to overheat.

Indeed, heat illness and hydration levels are integrally linked. But the nature of that link during running isn't as obvious as what medical experts have long thought. It turns out that the recommendation to drink, drink, and drink some more is a dangerous oversimplification. A new and unintended consequence arose among runners: what's known colloquially as "water intoxication" or "overhydration." The technical term for the condition is *hyponatremia,* and runners have actually died from it. According to Lewis Maharam, M.D., chairman of the International Marathon Medical Directors Association board of governors, hyponatremia is the most serious issue facing new and unconditioned distance runners.

What's happening. Hyponatremia means low blood sodium. It occurs when an athlete ingests so much water that sodium levels in the blood decrease dangerously. Confusion follows, organ function is impaired, and in severe cases, the condition can be life threatening.

Hyponatremia is sometimes exacerbated because the symptoms are easily mistaken for those of dehydration and heat illness: confusion, dizziness, headache, nausea, cramping, lack of coordination, and fatigue. Victims of hyponatremia have been encouraged (with disastrous results) to drink even more water or have been given fluid intravenously, placing them in more serious peril. How could such a seemingly benign and helpful piece of guidance be so misleading?

The rather sudden appearance of hyponatremia cases in distance-running races has been linked to the growing phenomenon in the past decade of relatively untrained runners training for the marathon and even greater distances. Most cases of hyponatremia occur on runs of a fairly slow pace that last in excess of 4 to 5 hours. Women, who comprise much of the ranks of newcomers to the sport, suffer the condition more often than men.

Researchers hypothesize that such very long, very slow runs by runners who have been admonished to drink regularly have created prime conditions for hyponatremia. Such runners, it turns out, are not producing tremendous amounts of body heat because of their slow pace; as a result, they are not generating copious amounts of sweat. Also, because of their slow pace, they are able to ingest greater amounts of liquid, often walking to get their fill during water stops. (Elite runners are exercising at a sufficiently intense degree that they are not able to ingest fluids efficiently, barely slowing their pace at water stops and typically swallowing only a few sips rather than an entire cupful.)

And why are women at greater risk? Because women tend to sweat less than men to begin with, and they have a lower body mass and smaller fluid requirements. On top of that, women tend to be the ones dutifully toting around their water bottles all day, obediently drinking what the doctor told them.

The problem sometimes is compounded in race situations by well-meaning volunteers and medical personnel who believe they are witnessing symptoms of dehydration and heat illness when a runner stumbles weakly into an aid station.

Running's major medical associations finally are addressing the risk of hyponatremia. Accordingly, the medical community is rethinking its stand on running and fluid intake. Race directors have been urged to decrease the number of water stations on their courses. Medical personnel have been told to no longer assume that runners must be suffering from dehydration and treated with an IV. "When we think someone may be hyponatremic, the emergency med techs are not to give an IV until sodium levels are checked," Dr. Maharam says.

What to do. In 2001 the International Marathon Medical Directors Association (IMMDA) took a major step back from the "drink as much as possible" paradigm. The official statement outlines the dangers of hyponatremia for the average runner and sets a recommended *upper* limit of fluid ingestion, instead of a minimum.

They recommend drinking no more than 400 to 800 milliliters (that's 13.3 to 26.6 ounces) per hour of exertion. The higher levels are for faster or heavier runners competing in warm conditions, the lower levels for slower runners in cooler conditions.

Still, any formula that attempts to spell out exactly how much each runner should drink per hour or mile is at best an estimate. Each runner's requirements are different, changing with variables such as weight, gender, weather, and conditioning. In addition, most runners won't have a reliable measure of how much they are consuming on the run anyway.

Significantly, the IMMDA also makes a point of saying that a runner is probably best served by the simplest formula there could be: paying attention to thirst.

Thirst had been getting a bad rap as an unreliable and lagging indicator of one's hydration level. ("By the time you're thirsty, it's too late," went the old thinking.) But the IMMDA statement turned that thinking on its head, recommending drinking "ad lib," which is to say, according to one's desires: "Several recent studies show that drinking *ad libitum* is as effective a drinking strategy during exercise as is drinking at the much higher rates proposed."

It's still very important for runners to understand the dangers of dehydration, and drinking to replenish lost fluids is crucial. But new research overwhelmingly shows that intentional overdrinking can be just as dangerous as not drinking at all. "If you drink by thirst, you'll drink enough.

If you drink more than that, you're overdrinking," concludes Dr. Maharam.

Of course, there's the flip side of the hydration equation. Some very fit runners feel invincible when it comes to heat and hydration. They believe that their high level of conditioning affords them the ability to run for miles and hours without drinking. While fitness and acclimation do make runners more efficient at dispersing heat, they do not make anyone immune to the effects of dehydration.

Conditioned runners will indeed feel fewer effects of heat and high humidity: They tend to be leaner and require less exertion to run than overweight, out-of-shape people. Conditioned athletes also tend to spill fewer electrolytes in their sweat (their sweat is less concentrated due to acclimation), so their requirements for both fluid and electrolytes might be less than those of "normal" people.

On the other hand, the more conditioned you are, the more you sweat, since your body becomes more efficient at cooling itself. That means overall fluid loss is greater.

WHEN AND WHAT TO DRINK

Here's what the latest guidelines from the International Marathon Medical Directors Association boil down to.

• Most runners do not need to drink any liquid on the run for sessions of less than 30 minutes. Drinking according to thirst before and after is fine.

• For runs between 30 minutes and an hour, novice runners might want to bring along a bottle of sports drink to sip on. Runners with at least a year of training behind them should have a sense of whether they can make it through the run comfortably with no additional fluids.

• Every runner should have fluids available for runs of more than 1 hour.

• Try to avoid plain water and instead consume a sports drink, which will replenish electrolytes.

• When on the run, drink enough to satisfy your thirst, but do not intentionally overdrink.

PROTECTION FROM THE SUN

Long hours outside mean that runners tend to be exposed to plenty of sun. And sun exposure is a proven risk for skin cancer. Runners should take precautions whenever possible by the following means.

• Run before 10:00 A.M. or after 5:00 P.M. The sun's rays are strongest at midday.

• Wear a full-spectrum sunscreen. Look for a lotion that is highly water resistant, so it doesn't wash off with your sweat. Also, look for formulas that contain zinc oxide, which provides a physical (not just chemical) barrier to the sun and has been shown to be most effective at blocking the sun.

• Slather on your sunblock lotion liberally. Studies have shown that most people don't use nearly enough lotion to provide the maximum level of protection. To cover your body fully, use roughly the amount that would fit in a shot glass.

• Wear a baseball cap. You can't put sunscreen on your hair, and your hair doesn't provide 100 percent protection for your scalp. Wearing a hat provides additional protection for your head and partially shades your face. Better yet, wear a cap with flaps that also cover your neck.

• Wear glasses that provide full-spectrum protection by screening the sun's rays. Long-term sun exposure has been linked to degenerative eye disease. When choosing sunglasses, check the label for information on sunblocking effectiveness: The darkness of the lenses does not indicate the level of protection they offer. For the strongest level of protection, look for the rating "Special Purpose," which indicates a 99 to 100 percent blockage of UVA and UVB radiation. "General Use" indicates a 95 percent blockage of UVB rays and 60 percent of UVA. Stay away from glasses labeled "Cosmetic," which block only 70 percent of UVB radiation.

It's pretty much a given that faster runners will become somewhat dehydrated on long runs and races; they're running too hard to replace all the fluids they're losing.

"If you look at elite athletes, they may drink once or twice in the whole race, and they don't even drink the whole cup, just a sip and they dump the rest on their head," says marathon medical director Dr. Maharam. "They'll finish the race dehydrated, but they're fine."

The important thing for these runners is to be aware of their limits and any significant changes in the way their body feels, drinking when necessary on long runs and then hydrating fully when they are finished running. The bottom line is that no matter how swift or experienced, no runner is immune to the effects of dehydration.

RUNNING IN THE COLD

Hypothermia and frostbite are the two most serious problems facing a runner in cold weather.

Hypothermia

Hypothermia is a sneaky condition. It is most dangerous when it creeps up on runners when they're least expecting it, usually in seemingly mild temperatures.

When the weather is truly cold, most runners dress for the part. You break out cozy cold-weather tights and jackets, cover your head, and pull on mittens. There's little chance that if you're this well-prepared, you'll be at risk for hypothermia—on an average run, you'll generate significant heat, and since you are dressed appropriately, you'll retain that heat.

It's the cool-but-not-cold fall or spring day, with temperatures in the 50s, when hypothermia can show up suddenly and unannounced. These are the days when you tend to be dressed in shorts and a T-shirt, no gloves, maybe just a baseball cap or nothing at all covering your head.

It's a day like this when, on a run of long duration, you might slow your pace as you tire. Suddenly, you're not generating as much body heat, and your scant clothing is little protection as body temperature begins to drop. Maybe the breeze has picked up, too, or rain begins to fall, cooling the body even more. Now you're at real risk of hypothermia, though temperatures never drop even close to freezing. Light cotton

WHY YOU NEED TO WARM UP

Warming up is never quite as important for runners as in cold weather. Muscle pulls are more likely in the cold, and other minor injuries, aches, and pains are more likely to become aggravated than in warm weather.

And by warming up, I don't mean stretching. Studies have shown that stretching cold muscles can actually *cause* injury. The best way to warm up in the cold is to jog very slowly for a few hundred yards, gradually limbering up your muscles. Then run the first mile of your workout at a slower pace than normal. After this point, you can transition into your regular pace. Or, if you are doing a faster run or tempo workout, this is the time to stop for a few minutes to stretch safely, but don't linger too long or you'll start to cool off.

Finally, realize that you probably won't be able to maintain as fast a pace as you could in more moderate temperatures. Cold weather means that your muscles will not be as limber and your body will be tensed against the cold, both of which slow your pace.

clothing that felt comfortable in the early miles now offers little protection against the elements.

What's happening. Hypothermia is generally diagnosed when body temperature drops below 97 degrees. It sets in when the body cannot generate enough heat fast enough to replace the heat it is losing to external conditions. Moisture and wind increase the risk of hypothermia, since both cool the body even further.

Early symptoms of hypothermia can include weakness, stumbling, chills, shivering, and confused speech and action. If the condition progresses, shivering (a warming mechanism) might cease. Left untreated, hypothermia can be fatal.

What to do. Prevent hypothermia by always wearing or bringing extra layers when you're planning on running an hour or more on cold and even cool days. (Hypothermia can occur when temperatures are in the 50s and even 60s.) A thin outer layer that can protect against sudden rain, snow, or wind can fold up and fit in a fanny pack. Also bring a hat, gloves, and long pants or tights. For everything from shirts to socks, wear wool and synthetics, which are preferable to cotton, since they retain their insulating properties even when damp.

A runner suffering from the early signs of hypothermia should take action immediately, depending on what resources are available. When possible, replace damp clothes with warm, dry clothes. Sip warm liquids. If there's a warm building nearby, get inside out of the chilly conditions.

Frostbite

You might feel impervious to frostbite when you run because the activity generates so much heat and you're generally not outside for prolonged periods of time. On long runs, however, you can be at risk. While actual frostbite is fairly rare for runners, frost-nip, a preliminary and less severe cold injury, is a more common warning.

What's happening. During prolonged exposure to cold, the body diverts blood toward the crucial organs. This leaves your extremities—fingers, toes, nose, ears—at risk. Even if you feel warm in your core area, you can get frostbite if your extremities are not covered. When frostbite sets in, actual ice crystals form in the body tissue. The skin typically first appears white, then red and swollen.

What to do. As with all other heat and cold injuries, prevention is the best medicine. When running in sub-freezing temperatures:

• Always wear a hat that covers your ears.

• Wear mittens, which retain body heat better than gloves. If you know you have poor circulation in your hands, use warming packs, sold at sporting goods and outdoor stores, and tuck these into your mittens.

• Wear thicker-than-usual wool or synthetic (rather than cotton) socks. You may need to buy a winter pair of running shoes half a size larger to accommodate your thicker socks; if your shoes are too tight, this will cut circulation to the area, exacerbating the risk of frostbite.

• In the coldest temperatures, if you plan to be out for a very long run, consider covering your face. A synthetic neck gaiter can be pulled up and worn over the lower half of your face, from your nose down. Some runners will wear balaclavas—full-face coverings with cutouts for nose, eyes, and mouth—but only the most severe cold temperatures warrant this type of intense protection.

• If you lose sensation in your fingers, toes, or ears while running, cut your run short and get inside. Warm yourself under a blanket or with additional clothes. Run comfortably warm water over the affected area.

In most cases, runners will suffer only frost-nip, a whitening of the skin that might eventually peel. If you suspect actual frostbite, see a doctor, who can determine the extent of tissue damage, clean and bandage the area, and prescribe antibiotics if necessary.

Finally, be sure that when you run in the cold you are well-hydrated before you set out. Because frostbite results from lack of bloodflow to the extremities, it can be exacerbated by dehydration, which reduces your blood volume, further limiting bloodflow.

WHAT YOU CAN DO

In very cold weather, details count. Follow these tips for cold-weather dressing to keep you comfortable on your runs.

Choose the right fabrics. Synthetic fabrics intended specifically for cold-weather running are worth the price. These materials draw sweat away from your body, helping you to retain an even body temperature. Stay away from cotton, which holds moisture and will end up cold and clammy against your skin.

Cover your head. Runners can lose much of their body heat through their heads. Synthetics work well; if you choose wool, look for a smooth band of material around your forehead area to prevent itching.

Wear mittens instead of gloves. Fingers stay warmer when they're together. Some runners prefer to layer a light pair of windproof mittens over a thin pair of running gloves.

Wear wool or synthetic blend socks. Once again, cotton is not your friend in cold weather. Wool and synthetic socks will keep your feet warm and dry even in wet conditions.

Use hand-warming packs. Runners who suffer from chronically cold hands due to poor circulation can use tiny disposable hand-warming packets, typically sold at outdoors and camping stores. Simply open a pair and tuck them in your mittens.

8

I'M INJURED. NOW WHAT?

TREATING THE MOST COMMON RUNNING INJURIES

I t's surprising how many runners meekly follow the ostrich approach to injury: They bury their heads in the sand, ignore the pain, and hope everything will miraculously turn out okay. Well, that's not how it works. Many injuries are minor at the onset but become more complicated with time and continued trauma.

TAKE ACTION

The best time to treat your running pain or injury is immediately. Not tomorrow. Not next week. Take action *as soon as* you notice all is not right with your body. Taking action means following several steps, the specifics of which will change depending on the nature of the injury. We'll address specific injuries and their treatment in the second half of this chapter. Meanwhile, early self-treatment for most injuries should entail a battle plan something like this.

Stop running. Or at least decrease your running intensity while you evaluate the situation.

Rest has gotten a bad rap. In a pendulum swing from the old days when all runners were admonished to stop exercising at the sight of a bruised toenail, runners today want to "train through" injury, no matter how agonizing.

The controversy over rest stems from the fact that taking time off from running rarely cures anything in and of itself. Rest offers only a partial, short-term solution to overuse injuries. Pain subsides temporarily, but when you start running again without treating the real cause of the problem (a biomechanical inefficiency, perhaps, or the wrong pair of shoes), pain resumes. Which is to say, time off from running does not solve the *underlying cause* of most overuse injuries.

But here's the other side of the story. Rest might not cure your injury, but it can relieve flaring symptoms of both overuse injuries and more acute injuries such as muscle strains. That's because stopping the repetitive forces for a few days or weeks (depending on the severity of the injury) can help inflammation subside and allow healing to start.

While some doctors will tell you it's okay to continue running while you heal, orthopedic surgeon Philip Stull, M.D., who specializes in treating professional athletes in Denver, questions the wisdom of training during the healing process. Running more won't always cause "outrageous damage," says Dr. Stull. But it will prolong healing. "If part of the problem is overuse, it doesn't make sense to go out and do it."

Besides, the fitness benefits you derive from severely curtailed training are minimal. Weigh the pros (minor fitness maintenance, some sanity savings) against the cons (continued trauma to the injury site). You can see why it might make sense just to take a week off altogether, rather than jog an easy 20 minutes every day—just enough to keep aggravating the injury site. Instead, Dr. Stull strongly recommends cross-training during the healing process to maintain fitness. "A lot of it comes down to common sense," Dr. Stull says. "Listen to your body—that's why God gave you nerve endings."

Those nerve endings provide the simplest way to know when you should stop running and take a break. "The golden rule is you should not run through pain," says Irene McClay Davis, Ph.D., an expert in biomechanics and a research director at Joyner Sports Medicine Institute in Newark, Delaware. "If you continue to run through pain, you develop compensatory strategies." The change in your stride might be subtle or even imperceptible, she says, but rest assured that it will result in other problems.

Not running through pain is a good rule of thumb, especially for beginners who have not lived through a spate of injuries and learned to read their bodies closely. We're talking about pain that feels worse and is much more specific than the general, next-day muscle soreness that results from healthy training, or other minor discomforts. If a new, sharp pain grows noticeable on a run, don't head out any farther; instead return home walking or at a slow jog, if that's comfortable.

Runners also need to take into account pain that makes itself known any time other than when you're running: in the morning, for example,

TO RUN OR NOT TO RUN

That's the question when you're hurt. And there's no easy answer. Here's a summary to help you decide whether to go for an easy jog (nothing more than that when you're hurting) or to proceed directly to a sports physician.

RUN . . .

• When you're feeling muscle aches that are not highly localized but are more general in nature
• When the pain subsides as you run—but also does not return in more severe fashion after you finish (Running masks some injuries because it can loosen tight fibers. The pain subsides temporarily but gets worse with each passing day. This is not an acceptable pattern, and it's best in this case to stop running in order to heal.)

DON'T RUN . . .

• When you are experiencing a stabbing, wincing pain
• When the pain clearly forces you to limp or otherwise alter your stride
• When the pain grows worse upon running
• When pain is evident at night or upon walking as well as running
• When range of motion is obviously reduced or there is visible trauma such as severe swelling

or when walking down stairs. It can be difficult to make the connection between such pain and your running, but there's a good chance your running is the culprit. Just because the pain subsides during exercise doesn't mean you don't have a running injury. Many injuries subside specifically during the run—due to increased bloodflow and endorphins—only to roar back afterward. If the general trend is that your pain increases with each run, then that's reason to take a break.

If you've caught your injury early, a few days off might suffice to allow healing to begin. For the next few days, you're allowed to try to run, but only if you promise to back off and stop at the first sign of pain. Try jogging slowly. Cut back your distance. Forgo any hilly routes. Run on a soft surface instead of pavement.

The idea is to test things out. If the pain resumes immediately, it's best not to run. If you can run slowly without pain, it's fine to jog easily for up to 30 minutes. But the most important rule of all is that you still must faithfully take action with the other steps below, treating your injury and determining the cause. Otherwise, all the rest in the world won't help.

Treat with PRICE. That stands for protection, rest, ice, compression, and elevation.

Many people are familiar with the standard RICE treatment. Some doctors now add the P for "protection" as a reminder not to do more damage to the site. This update on an old standby is a safe and reliable starting point for home treatment of many running injuries. That's because so many running pains involve an inflammation response with swelling, including tendinitis, muscle strains, runner's knee, shin splints, plantar fasciitis, and more.

PRICE works to decrease both inflammation and pain. In effect, you're helping the body reabsorb fluids that have pooled at the injury site. By drawing blood to the affected area, waste products are flushed away. That's important because swelling slows down the healing process. PRICE maximizes the environment for healing, explains Larry Grollman, director of sports medicine at the University of Pittsburgh Medical Center for Sports Medicine.

PRICE won't work for all injuries—stress fractures, for example—but this is an appropriate place to start self-treatment in many cases. Besides, it can never make things worse.

Here's a closer look at each step of the process.

Protection. Protect the area so that it does not suffer further aggravation. Protection might include anything from an elastic bandage to crutches or just staying off your feet.

Rest. I discussed rest in the previous section. Rest can be relative: Your decision will be whether to continue running at a reduced level of intensity or to stop altogether for a few days. Remember, pain is your guide when making this decision. Also, rest should be your mantra throughout the whole day, not just during workout time. Limit other activities that stress the area. If walking or driving makes it hurt, then don't walk or drive if possible.

Ice. The best way to ice most injuries is to strap an ice pack to the site with an elastic bandage. (If you do this, you take care of the com-

DO'S AND DON'TS FOR ICING

DO . . .

• Ice the injured area for 10 to 20 minutes at a stretch; any longer can cause tissue damage.
• Ice immediately after a run or any other stress to the injury site. The sooner the inflammation is addressed, the more effective the ice will be.
• Ice at least twice a day and up to five times a day.
• Allow at least 1 hour between ice sessions, to let the injury site return to normal temperature.

DON'T . . .

• Use store-bought ice packs and wraps if possible. These warm rapidly with body heat, providing only a few moments of true icing effect. Instead, make an ice pack with ice cubes or crushed ice. Even a bag of frozen vegetables does the job.
• Run immediately after icing. Ice will tighten the area, making it inflexible and temporarily more prone to injury. Wait at least an hour if you must run after you've iced; better yet, reserve ice for *after* your runs.

pression and elevation steps at the same time. Simply sit or lie down to elevate the injury while your ice pack is strapped on.) Ice for 10 to 20 minutes at a stretch. Less than that amount of time is insufficient for the desired healing response, and more than that raises the risk of tissue injury at the site. Packs that are not already lined with some type of fabric should be wrapped in a thin cloth.

You can also give yourself an ice massage. Create a massager by freezing water in a Styrofoam cup. Then peel part of the cup away to expose the ice. Hold the rest of the ice with the remaining cup. This method is particularly useful for small tendinous areas. If you actively massage with ice, limit the time to 10 minutes at a stretch.

Compression. Wrap the area with an elastic bandage. It should be tight but not so much so that bloodflow is restricted. If pain or tingling results, the bandage is too tight. The exact wrapping technique will depend on the site, but in general you'll be circling the bandage around, aiming to compress the entire affected area.

Compression is intended to minimize swelling; it should not be used as a crutch to keep you running. For example, if your ankle is strained, many physical therapists believe it's best to allow the area to heal properly before running again. If you run with an ankle brace or tape job, muscles in the area can become lazy and eventually lose their strength and stabilizing ability.

Elevation. Whenever possible, elevate the injury above heart level to minimize swelling. You can do this when sitting at your desk, watching television, even sleeping.

Take anti-inflammatories, within reason. Pain relievers have a place in injury treatment. They can reduce inflammation and alleviate discomfort. Problems arise when runners depend on such medications to get them through a run or take the drugs in such great quantities that they cause other health problems.

The reality is, taking too much will not help you heal any faster or provide any preventive value. It might, however, aggravate your stomach—when taken in excess, anti-inflammatories can lead to ulcers. Always take the pills with a meal to minimize stomach irritation.

Taking an anti-inflammatory before a workout may dangerously mask pain signals that would otherwise warn you to stop running. Only after the drug wears off would you realize your mistake. Instead, take the medication after your run to reduce inflammation and damage when you are training through an injury or returning to running after an injury-induced break.

Finally, always use a true anti-inflammatory. In most cases, you want the anti-inflammatory properties of the medication, not only pain relief. Stick to the drugs that fall under the category of nonsteroidal anti-inflammatories (NSAIDs). These include aspirin and ibuprofen—which is sold under several brand names, including Advil and Motrin. Acetaminophen (Tylenol), while an effective painkiller, does not reduce swelling.

Schedule a doctor's appointment. See a doctor right away for an injury if:

• Pain is always present, even when you're walking or resting

• You have visible trauma (swelling, redness) and limited range of motion

• You believe you suffered an acute injury such as a fracture or a severe sprain

In most cases, however, running injuries are not this dramatic. Typically, you'll find yourself with a pain that allows you to try self-treatment in the manner outlined above.

If you've suffered a simple soft-tissue strain or a pull because of overly zealous training and you've been following the above steps—rest, PRICE, and anti-inflammatories—chances are you'll notice that the pain will subside more each day. After a few days, you might successfully have healed yourself.

If, on the other hand, you've done all of the above steps but the pain hasn't subsided within a week or so, then it's time to see a sports medicine specialist. In this case, your injury might be more complicated in nature. You might require a prescription for orthotics to adjust your biomechanics. You might require physical therapy to heal the trauma. In some rare cases, you might need surgery.

If you can see a sports physician rather than your general physician, do so. And if you can see a doctor who specializes in *running* injuries in particular versus other sports, that's even better.

Sports medicine clinics (and physicians) have proliferated across the country in recent years, giving recreational athletes access to top-notch treatment. That's great, but don't assume a practice fits your needs just because "sports" is printed on the sign out front. Many sports practices

WHAT'S IN A NAME?

In most cases, your family doctor is not the best person to see for a running injury. If options in your area are few, your general doctor can refer you to somebody else, but that will be about the extent of his expertise. You need a specialist who is familiar with treating running injuries.

There's no one right type of doctor that corresponds to each injury. In many cases, the precise professional you visit can be up to you. If you already have a relationship with a podiatrist, orthopedist, or physical therapist, you might want to start there. "It's the experience and reputation of the professional who's going to deliver the care that matters more than the initials after the name," says podiatrist Thomas Shonka, past president of the American Academy of Podiatric Sports Medicine. The only mandate is that the doctor understands the nature of your injury. "Go to somebody who understands and has experience in treating running injuries."

Here's a look at some of the specialists you might choose to see for your running injury and what each does.

Sports medicine physician. A general family physician who specializes in athletics. Devoted runners whose training is a priority will find such knowledge a comfort even in addressing nonrunning ailments. A sports medicine physician is a great place to start for most running injuries; he will know when to refer you to another specialist if necessary.

Podiatrist. Podiatrists specialize in care of the foot. They are not

specialize in standard team sports, and that's not going to help you. "Working with runners is different than treating a football player with a blown knee," Grollman says.

A sports physician who's used to treating football injuries views the knee as a self-contained unit. "In running," Grollman explains, "we're not just treating a knee. We're treating the whole body. If your patella hurts, we'll look at your back, hip, and ankle, too." A running specialist medical doctors. As you would with other practitioners, look for a podiatrist who further specializes in sports and, ideally, running. Podiatrists treat foot injuries, analyze running gait, and craft orthotics. If your pain resides in the foot or ankle, a podiatrist who specializes in running is a good place to start your treatment.

Orthopedist. This is a surgeon who is trained to treat injuries to both muscles and bones and their connective tissues, including ligaments, cartilage, and tendons. Because of the possibility of complications, runners should exhaust all other noninvasive avenues before resorting to surgery for a running injury.

Chiropractor. A practitioner who manipulates the spine and joints to restore proper functioning and range of movement and to alleviate pain. (See chapter 9 for more on chiropractic.)

Physical therapist. He's not a doctor but is trained in the working mechanics of the body. Physical therapists specialize in injury rehabilitation and prevention, typically working with the runner to develop a program of strengthening and flexibility. Many insurance companies require a referral from a physician in order to cover a physical therapist's services. Traditionally, athletes would see physical therapists after conferring with a doctor. Now many runners are seeking out the services of a sports physical therapist sooner in the injury process, particularly for soft-tissue strains that can benefit from modalities such as ultrasound and electrical stimulation.

also will know to look at your full body's biomechanics while you're actually running, not just walking. And he'll know to ask you about your running history and whether you've recently changed your shoes or increased your mileage.

Find a running specialist through word of mouth. Ask your training partners, call your local running club or coaches, go to a running specialty store. Someone in town will likely be known as "the runners' doctor." That's who you want to see. Start with a sports medicine physician who treats runners, if one is available. If your pain is located in your foot, it's also okay to start with a podiatrist who focuses on runners. Either type of physician will then refer you to an orthopedist, physical therapist, or other specialist if necessary.

Once you find a practice, don't wait for an appointment if you can help it. If you get a time slot several days or weeks out, ask to get on the waiting list in case there's a cancellation. They can almost always squeeze you in earlier. If you have an overuse injury and pain has been building slowly, it's probably not fair to weasel your way onto the appointment book immediately. But if you suffered an acute injury, let the nurse or receptionist know and you might get into one of their emergency slots.

Whomever you see, you'll want to walk away feeling certain that the underlying cause of your injury has been addressed so that you minimize the risk of it happening again. If your foot hurts, it's not enough to alleviate the pain. You and your doctor together must determine why it hurt

WHAT THE PROS KNOW

TAKE CHARGE OF YOUR HEALTH

Studies have shown that patients who ask questions and are informed about their health problems receive better care. It's no different with running injuries. By being aggressive about your treatment, you ensure that you get proper diagnosis and care and possibly heal faster.

Being aggressive doesn't mean bullying the receptionist or disputing your doctor's every word. It just means playing an active role in your own care and taking responsibility for your healing. Become an "expert" on your injury. Read this and other books, check the Internet, talk with running friends. Inform yourself of treatments that have worked for others. Outline your questions before you see your specialist. And before you leave the doctor's office, ask questions and write down the answers, if necessary. If you don't understand any of the medical jargon, ask the doctor to clarify it for you.

in the first place, then treat the cause with strengthening, stretching, a change of shoes, or some other course of action. If you've suffered a stress fracture, your doctor should order a check of your bone density and, depending on the results, perhaps even send you to a nutritionist. If you're told to wait for the bone to knit and sent on your way, that's not adequate treatment. Without knowing the reason behind your injury, you risk a recurrence as soon as you start running again.

Any time you have nagging doubts after leaving a doctor's office, it's worth getting another opinion. If you feel your concerns weren't addressed, for example, or the doctor couldn't find the root cause of your pain, or you were advised to simply stop running, it's time to see another specialist.

COMING BACK FROM INJURY

When you resume running after a break or reduced training intensity, let pain be your guide. It's okay to run as long as your pain is subsiding rather than getting worse with each passing day.

Your body will feel different than it did before you stopped running. You might feel awkward if you haven't run at all for several days or weeks. You might have gained some weight. You might feel out of shape and out of breath. That's okay. You'll regain your fitness, and patience is your key to a successful return.

Some injury sites will feel different than they did before, even after they're fully healed. Pay close attention to how they feel to avoid reinjuring the area. The irony is that sometimes it's necessary to run through discomfort on your way back to fitness, particularly in the case of muscle strains and injuries involving connective tissue.

During the healing process, adhesions (or scar tissue) sometimes form around the injury site. According to Mark Plaatjes, a former elite runner who is now a physical therapist at In Motion Rehabilitation in Boulder, Colorado, active people often have an abundance of collagen, a protein that is formed during healing. Their bodies do too good a job healing, and the excess protein "acts like superglue." This means even healthy fibers can be bound up with adhesions.

When this scar tissue forms around the injury, you might feel a tightness or a slight tugging sensation. This doesn't mean that you can't run, but you do need to monitor the level of discomfort. If pain decreases with each day's run, you're on the right track. If pain is growing around the injury site, you need to revisit your treatment and see the physician again—and don't increase your training yet.

Here are a few additional guidelines for returning to your running routine after an injury-induced break.

Follow the "laws of training and injury." Build gradually and incrementally from your starting point. You cannot rush the fitness process—running too much, too soon will only result in new aches and pains. (See chapter 2.)

Add distance (or time) first and intensity later. Run easy before you run hard, since fast running creates more impact and stress on the body. For the same reason, run on flat ground for several days or even weeks before you run hills. Rebuild your base of easy distance runs before you attempt intervals or tempo runs.

Stay close to home. For the first few days of training, run a short loop or go out and back, never straying too far. This way if pain flares up, you're only a short jog or walk from home or your car. If you head out for a full 20 minutes and then find yourself in trouble, you'll have a long walk home. This might further aggravate your injury, and you might be tempted to keep jogging just to get back faster.

Visit a massage therapist. A good time to visit a sports massage therapist is around the same time you return to training, particularly after soft-tissue injuries. Intense bodywork can help to break up collagen adhesions (scar tissue) and ensure that other muscles stay loose and healthy as you resume stressing your body with training. (For more on massage, see chapter 9.)

Break out a new pair of shoes. Old shoes might have contributed to your original injury. Even if that's not the case, you'll need extra protection when you resume running. If there's any doubt in your mind as to whether you need new shoes, err on the side of caution: Recycle the old ones and invest in your health with a new pair.

THE MOST COMMON RUNNING INJURIES

Running ailments take all forms, of course, and some are obscure and difficult to diagnose. But many of the aches and pains runners suffer fall into one of the categories described in the remainder of this chapter.

GETTING TO THE ROOT
OF THE PROBLEM

This chapter focuses on healing running injuries once they've occurred. Think of this in two distinct ways.

• Healing the actual trauma so you can return to running without pain
• Determining the underlying cause of your injury to prevent recurrence

Most runners ignore the second part in an effort to patch up their ills and hurry out the door for a run. But without identifying the root causes of injury, relapse is almost certain. In fact, about half of all running injuries are considered recurrences. Half. That means runners would save themselves a lot of trouble if they took the time to learn from their problems the first time around.

So don't stop once you've iced and ibuprofened your way back to training. Continue your detective work—with the assistance of a trained sports medicine professional—to determine what strengthening and stretching you need to do or what changes you need to make to your footwear. Keep yourself from becoming part of the recurrence statistic.

The advice for treatment you see here is offered after interviews with many prominent sports medicine professionals. Chief among them are podiatrist Thomas Shonka, past president of the American Academy of Podiatric Sports Medicine, and orthopedic surgeon Philip Stull.

You might notice that the recommended course of action for many of these injuries looks similar. That's because many of these injuries are due to overuse and therefore can be addressed early in their course with a combination of some common sense, at-home treatment, and thorough evaluation of biomechanics by a sports medicine professional.

Ankle Sprain

What you feel. Ankle sprains can range from mild to excruciating. Intense pain might be accompanied by an audible pop when the injury occurs. Sometimes, pain subsides quickly and is replaced by general soreness. In more serious cases, pain remains severe and is accompanied by inflammation and tenderness around the injury site.

Cause. One of the few acute injuries that runners experience, an ankle sprain is usually caused by a misstep—off a curb, over a rock, into a hole. The ankle rolls excessively on one side or the other, tugging or tearing the ligaments in the area.

Treatment:

• If pain and swelling are severe, see a doctor to determine if any bones have broken.

• PRICE it: Use protection, rest, ice, compression, and elevation (see page 96).

• Take an anti-inflammatory like aspirin or ibuprofen.

• Discontinue running while pain is severe. Let pain be your guide as you return to running. While you needn't be entirely pain-free to resume training, do not run if you are limping or if running makes the pain worse.

• Use ankle tape and braces sparingly and only in the acute phase of injury. Tape and braces should not be worn to get through a run. Support systems such as these used to be recommended to keep an athlete from reinjuring the ankle. More recent research has shown that such immobilization can become a crutch, weakening surrounding musculature and detracting from a person's ability to control his own ankle mobility.

• As soon as pain subsides, exercise with resistance tubing and/or a wobble board to help rehabilitate the site. Such

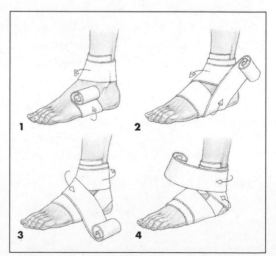

ANKLE-TAPING TECHNIQUE

Follow the arrows in each picture for proper ankle-wrapping technique. Wrap your ankle only during the most acute phase of your injury.

strength and flexibility exercises are important because an ankle weakened from one sprain is more susceptible to future injury.

To use resistance tubing, anchor it around a sturdy object. Loop the other end of the tubing around the injured foot. Sit on the floor facing the point of resistance with your legs straight out in front of you so that you feel slight resistance. Flex your foot against the point of resistance, pulling it back toward your body, to the left, and to the right.

Wobble boards—which vary in design but generally feature a platform with a round-shaped bottom—can be purchased in most sporting goods stores. The goal is simply to stand on the board and work to stay upright, without letting the platform tip over to one side. The exercise develops the small muscles in the foot, ankle, and lower leg, improving not only strength but also balance and reaction time.

Healing time. A few days up to several weeks.

Compartment Syndrome

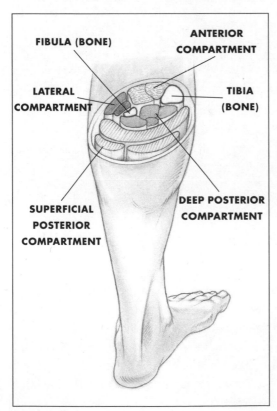

FIBULA (BONE)

ANTERIOR COMPARTMENT

LATERAL COMPARTMENT

TIBIA (BONE)

DEEP POSTERIOR COMPARTMENT

SUPERFICIAL POSTERIOR COMPARTMENT

What you feel. Pain in the calf that comes on gradually during running but can become very severe. Tingling or numbness in the foot or toes is also possible, but most runners will be forced to stop before reaching this point. Pain typically stops with cessation of running.

Cause. Muscles in the lower leg are divided into four compartments that are contained by fascia, a sheath of connective tissue. In compartment syndrome,

LEG COMPARTMENTS

Your lower-leg muscles reside in four compartments underneath a layer of connective tissue.

increased fluid from exertion can swell the area to such a critical degree that bloodflow is impeded and nerves are compressed.

Compartment syndrome actually is rare among recreational runners (elite runners are more apt to have overdeveloped their muscles to the degree that makes swelling more likely). However, the symptoms can be confused with those of a stress fracture or shin splints and, for that reason, warrant explanation in this section.

Treatment. This is one of the few running injuries that virtually always requires surgical intervention. A runner can stop running, administer ice massage, and take oral anti-inflammatories, and the pain will likely abate, only to return when running is resumed.

An orthopedist can confirm a diagnosis of compartment syndrome with a treadmill test. The athlete runs until pain develops, then the physician inserts a needle to test the pressure in the muscle compartment. Once the diagnosis is confirmed, the physician will perform a *fasciotomy*, in which the fascia is cut to relieve the pressure in the compartment.

Healing time. After a fasciotomy: 2 to 4 weeks.

Groin Pain

Groin pain is most typically due to muscle strain and sometimes due to stress fracture of a bone in the pubic area. These can sometimes be distinguished by the onset of symptoms: A strain will develop gradually and be more diffuse, while a stress fracture will present itself more suddenly and be localized. However, a visit to the doctor for confirmation of diagnosis is recommended. For more information, see the sections in this chapter on "Muscle Strains and Tears" and "Stress Fractures."

Iliotibial (IT) Band Syndrome

What you feel. Sharp pain on the outside of the kneecap. Pain typically presents itself during a run and disappears once the run is finished. Pain is often more noticeable when you're running downhill.

Cause. Tightness and/or inflammation of the IT band, connective tissue that runs along the outside of the leg, connecting the hip to the inside of the knee. IT band flare-ups are typically due to training overload, either in terms of overall mileage or speedwork. Contributing factors can include underpronation, weakness in the hip abductor muscles, and running on slanted or downhill surfaces. The pain is due to the tugging of the band at the knee connection, but treatment must target the runner's overall biomechanics.

Treatment:

- Take an anti-inflammatory like aspirin or ibuprofen.

- Apply ice at the pain site.

- Reduce training intensity. That means no running at all for several days to avoid further inflammation. Most cross-training should be avoided as well, including any activity that flexes the knee joint. Swimming—using only the arms and immobilizing the legs—is acceptable. When treatment begins to reduce the pain, you can slowly phase easy jogging back in.

- Evaluate your shoes. You might need shoes that provide greater cushioning. Consult a sports physician for a biomechanical evaluation, if necessary.

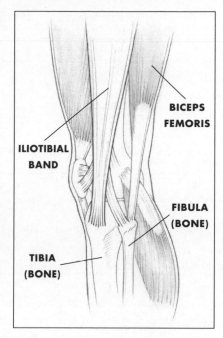

ILIOTIBIAL BAND

The iliotibial band connects the hip to the inside of your knee.

- Seek massage or physical therapy. A trained sports therapist can target trigger points, encourage flexibility, and reduce pain.

- Engage in a full-body stretching program at least once a day. Focus particularly on the legs, hips, and buttocks. (See stretches in chapter 4.) While the IT band itself does not stretch, it's important to maintain flexibility in the muscles to which it is related.

- Correct imbalances. If pain persists, a sports doctor or physical therapist can prescribe specific strengthening exercises to correct imbalances that have contributed to the IT band syndrome.

- Rehabilitation treatment resolves most cases successfully. Surgery is an extremely rare necessity and should be considered only in cases in which aggressive rehabilitation has failed.

Healing time. Several weeks.

Muscle Strains and Tears

What you feel. Sensation that ranges from a twinge or tightness to a severe, debilitating pain, typically localized in a specific area of one muscle. Pain becomes worse with use of the muscle or upon applying pressure to the site. The most typical sites runners strain are the hamstring and groin area, but almost any area can be injured in this manner.

Cause. Except for sprinters, runners don't typically suffer acute muscle pulls. That's because a true, severe muscle tear is caused by sudden, extreme exertion. Most distance runners, on the other hand, engage in moderate exercise that is fairly constant and far gentler in terms of effort. Even during track workouts, recreational distance runners do not engage in truly explosive running.

Distance runners do suffer muscle damage, however. These injuries could more accurately be called chronic muscle strains, and they are overuse injuries rather than acute events. In this case, muscle fibers in a specific location suffer repeated microtrauma. Continued strain and ensuing development of scar tissue in the area eventually create a weak, tender knot in the muscle. The runner doesn't technically have a torn hamstring, but he does have an aggravated, debilitated one.

Treatment:

• Ice the area, particularly after a session of massage or physical therapy.

• Evaluate your training and cut back on excessive long runs or fast workouts until pain subsides.

• Visit a trained massage therapist or physical therapist who specializes in treating runners. He will perform cross-friction fiber work, a rigorous, deep-tissue massage that breaks up adhesions in the area caused by excessive scar tissue. This will help the muscle fibers return to their proper form and functioning. This can be an excruciating process but will reduce pain in the long run. Acupuncture also can be effective. (See chapter 9 for more on acupuncture.)

• When pain subsides, engage in an extensive flexibility program. Do not, however, stretch the area when the muscle is actively strained and painful, since this can tear more of the weakened muscle fibers. (See chapter 4 for more information on stretching.)

Healing time. Several days (if caught very early) to several weeks. However, once aggravated, muscle strains tend to recur, sometimes over the course of years. Repeat the treatment process each time pain is again noticeable in the affected area.

Plantar Fasciitis

What you feel. Upon impact, an aching, localized pain underneath the heel of the foot. Pain is most severe after inactivity; for example, first thing in the morning. If left to progress, the pain from plantar fasciitis can become so severe that it makes even walking unbearable.

Cause. Excess movement in the event of overpronation can cause tugging on the plantar fascia, a swath of connective tissue that runs along the bottom of the foot, where it connects to the heel bone. Trauma at the site causes pain and inflammation; eventually, a bone spur can develop from scarring at the site.

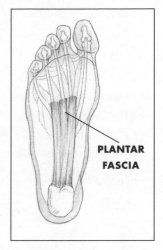

PLANTAR FASCIA

The plantar fascia runs along the bottom of your foot from your toes to the heel bone.

Treatment:

• Take an anti-inflammatory like aspirin or ibuprofen.

• Discontinue or severely curtail your training for at least a few days while figuring out your course of treatment. Cross-train with non-impact activities (swimming, water running) until you can run pain-free without limping. Resume running very gradually and only after you have followed the next steps to ensure you are wearing proper footwear.

• Have a sports medicine professional examine your biomechanics by watching you run and walk on a treadmill.

• Purchase motion-control shoes and/or orthotics to correct excessive pronation.

• Wear shoes with proper support at all times, not just during runs. Walking barefoot around the house or wearing flimsy shoes such as flip-flops can delay healing.

• In severe cases, a doctor might recommend a cortisone injection; such treatment is considered generally safe in this area of the foot.

• Stretch your calf muscles (see page 50). Pay particular attention to your foot position while stretching to ensure that you are not exacerbating the tugging of the fascia: Keep your foot in the supinated position—rolled to the outside instead of letting it flop inward at the ankle. This is critical because if your foot rolls in, you're not really stretching your calf area but stretching and tugging the fascia. The supinated position does not stress the fascia, and the stretch occurs at the proper site in the calf.

• Some runners find relief from pain with the use of a night splint. This device holds the foot in a flexed position overnight, thus eliminating trauma to the site that can occur when the first steps of the day restretch and tug the injury site.

• Surgical or other intervention is required in only a very small percentage of cases. The latest treatment is shock-wave therapy, in which the attachment area of the fascia is blasted with shock waves up to 2,000 times a session. Done under anesthesia on an outpatient basis, the treatment creates an inflammatory response that leads to the development of new blood vessels in the area, thus promoting healing.

Healing time. Four weeks to several months.

Runner's Knee (Patellofemoral Pain Syndrome)

What you feel. Pain around the kneecap that tends to originate and intensify during runs. As the injury progresses, pain also might be felt when sitting with legs bent or when climbing or descending stairs.

Cause. The pain is a result of improper tracking of the knee, specifically of the patella (kneecap), as it glides up and down in the femoral groove. This deviation is usually due to some anatomical problem, such as excessive pronation, leg-length discrepancy, muscle imbalance, or iliotibial band tightness. Early in the injury, the pain is due to irritation at the kneecap; left to progress, actual deterioration of the knee cartilage can occur.

Treatment:

• Apply ice at the pain site. Again, this can temporarily relieve the pain but does not solve the underlying problem.

• Take an anti-inflammatory like aspirin or ibuprofen.

• Get a thorough analysis of your gait and biomechanics from a running health specialist. He will recommend proper shoes and possibly orthotics to correct anatomical inefficiencies. Customized orthotics might be necessary for very mobile feet, since the inserts provide support superior to over-the-counter models.

• The evaluation should include an assessment of quadriceps strength. Depending on those results, your physician or therapist might prescribe strengthening exercises.

• Replace worn-out or inappropriate shoes with motion-control shoes.

• Reduce training intensity until pain subsides. Eliminate speed and hill workouts temporarily. Rest helps heal trauma to the area and helps reduce pain but does not actually treat the cause. Once you resume running, if you haven't analyzed your gait and purchased proper shoes or shoe inserts, the problem and the pain will resume.

Healing time. Several weeks to several months.

Shin Splints

What you feel. Pain or aching that develops slowly in the lower leg. At first, it is possible to run through the pain, but if ignored, shin pain can become severe enough so that you have to discontinue training.

Cause. The causes of shin pain are numerous. In fact, the term "shin splints" is not a medical diagnosis but a catchall phrase that refers to any type of pain between the knee and the ankle. Pain might be caused by bone trauma, muscle tears, tendinitis, or a combination of the three. And these are likely caused by overtraining errors, often compounded by incorrect shoe choice or worn-out shoes.

The most classic presentation of shin splints is now thought to be similar in nature to plantar fasciitis. As tension at the site develops, the sheath that holds the tendon in place can actually pull away the *periosteum,* or outer covering of the bone. "We used to think it was the muscle pulling away, but it's deep in the tendon," Dr. Shonka explains. If the protective bone covering is traumatized enough, a stress fracture can result.

Treatment:

• Use ice massage at the pain site.

• Take an anti-inflammatory like aspirin or ibuprofen.

• See a sports medicine professional when pain has persisted more than a week. Because shin splints can be caused by so many different factors, a visit to a sports medicine professional is required to determine the underlying problem. Self-treatment with rest and ice might alleviate pain temporarily, but unless the cause is determined, pain will return when regular training is resumed.

• Reduce training intensity until the cause is determined.

• Physical therapy treatments, such as ultrasound or electrical stimulation, can speed healing.

• New, appropriate shoes or orthotics might be ordered by your physician.

• Strength and flexibility exercises might be prescribed based on your biomechanics.

Healing time. A few weeks up to several months.

Stress Fractures

What you feel. Sharp, intense pain that is very localized. Typically the pain is so severe that you must stop running immediately. Some stress fractures present early warning signs of general pain, but most are felt suddenly. Stress fractures are most common in runners in the tibia and fibula (the large and small shinbones) and the metatarsal bones of the feet. Other possible sites include the femur, pubic and hip area, and ankle area.

Cause. Classic overtraining—running too much or too fast when the body is not conditioned appropriately. Contributing factors can be running on hard surfaces and worn-out shoes that do not protect against shock.

Women in particular are prone to stress fractures if they suffer from low bone density due to poor nutrition and/or menstrual irregularities.

Treatment:

• See your sports physician immediately. Most stress fractures will not show up right away on an x-ray, but a qualified physician should be able to determine when a stress fracture is suspected. Subsequent x-rays, usually performed after a few weeks, or a bone scan will confirm healing at the site, which shows up as scar tissue where the bone has knit together.

• Complete rest is required for healing. Some doctors will have patients wear a cast—this is not so much to facilitate healing but to ensure that the site gets adequate rest.

• A bone density test and nutritional workup might be in order, particularly for women. If your bone density is low, boost your calcium intake. Both men and women should consume at least 1,000 milligrams of calcium daily. Women under the age of 25 or who are pregnant need 1,500 milligrams. The best food source for calcium is dairy products, including low-fat milk, yogurt, and cheese. Green vegetables, particularly broccoli and kale, are also excellent sources, as are fish, tofu, and fortified juice. Supplements can help ensure that women get enough calcium, but food sources are always preferable since they are absorbed better by the body and provide a variety of nutrients. Menopausal women should talk to their doctor about other measures to fend off bone loss. (For more on bone health in women, see chapter 13.)

• In many cases, the only appropriate cross-training is water running. Ask your doctor for a removable cast, which will allow access to the pool.

• Bone stimulation devices that speed healing might be available. However, these are very expensive and only occasionally covered by insurance. Bone stimulation is typically reserved for professional athletes or others whose livelihood depends on a speedy return to health.

• Resume training very gradually. Once you've taken time off for a stress fracture, your body will be deconditioned. Start your running program by alternating walking and running for brief periods, so that

(continued on page 118)

FOOT TROUBLE

They're not as serious as a sprained ankle or a stress fracture, but even minor foot problems sideline many runners. Here's how to handle some of the most common.

Blisters. Blisters are caused by friction or pressure, which causes layers of the skin to separate and fill with fluid. Properly fitting running shoes can help prevent them. The toe box should have enough room so that your feet don't jam against the front of the shoe. Sometimes, blisters are caused by new socks that bunch up in spots or don't provide enough sweat absorption on a long run.

You've probably been told never to pop blisters because of the risk of infection. If you're like most runners, you've probably also ignored this advice. If you insist on popping a minor blister to alleviate discomfort in order to run, at least follow these precautions.
• Use a sterile needle (sterilize it by holding a match to the needle until it turns red, but let it cool before you proceed).
• Pop it toward the outside edge and gently press out the liquid.
• Cover the blister with an antibiotic ointment and a bandage or medicated skin covering.
• Surround the blister (but do not cover it) with a layer of moleskin to minimize contact and pressure on the area.
• Wear different running shoes than the ones that caused the problem, so that you're not exerting pressure in the very same spot.
• When you're done running, wash the area well with soap and water and re-cover it.
• In the case of a large, angry blister that clearly interferes with your foot plant, don't even try to run. You'll be either aggravating the area or compensating with your stride. Take a few days to let the worst trauma heal.

Hammertoe. This is the term for toes that curl or buckle down permanently. Running can exacerbate the problem, especially if the runner repeatedly wears shoes that are too small or tight. The condition also can develop from ill-fitting or uncomfortable street shoes. Hammertoe is most common in the second toe—particularly when it is longer than the big toe—but some runners experience buckling in several toes. Pain and inflammation can develop on the tip of the toe.

Treatment primarily involves getting proper shoes. Runners should reevaluate all their footwear—street shoes and athletic shoes—to ensure they are the correct size. Shoes also can be supplemented with a pad cut to fit the area and reduce pressure on the site. In severe cases, surgery might be necessary to correct the situation. But this is a fairly drastic measure, and many runners find they are able to run through the condition without excessive pain.

Neuroma. A neuroma is an inflammation of the nerve. Sharp, localized pain is felt under or between the metatarsal bones (the long bones that make up the body of the foot) at the site of the affected nerve. Scar tissue at the site eventually creates a very tender knot, which becomes more difficult to treat as time passes.

Caught early, a neuroma might be successfully treated with padded shoe inserts that relieve pressure on the area or with an injection of anti-inflammatories. If scarring has progressed, however, surgery might be required to remove the knot of tissue.

Pain on top of the foot. Sometimes pain over the top of the foot can be caused by nothing more than tight shoelaces. If the pain is present only during running, try adjusting the lacing pattern and tightness of your running shoes to take pressure off the tender spot.

Pain in the area of the metatarsals that is present at all times might be an indication of a stress fracture. Typically, this pain will be very localized and so intense that it does not allow running. (See the "Stress Fractures" section on page 114.)

your bones, muscles, and connective tissue can all readapt to the impact of running without the onset of a new injury.

Healing time. Healing times vary depending on which bone is affected but generally take between 6 and 10 weeks.

Tendinitis of the Achilles

What you feel. Achilles tendinitis presents itself gradually. First the runner feels a general discomfort, pain that is present early in the day before walking or after a run when the leg has tightened up. As the condition progresses, however, the tendon (located above the heel and below the calf) will become painful to the touch in a specific spot and cause limping during running and even walking. Redness and inflammation will become visible in the tendon area. Upon movement of the tendon, a creaking sensation—sometimes described as the feeling of packing snow—will be apparent. Tendinitis can occur just about anywhere in the body, but in runners it is most commonly found in the Achilles.

Cause. Tendinitis is inflammation of the tendon caused by trauma to the area from overexertion—too many miles, too much speedwork, too many hills, or improper shoes that do not protect the foot and cause the tendon to overwork. If you don't address the cause and continue training, damage to the tendon can become so severe that the fibers tear, leading to a partial or complete rupture of the tendon.

Treatment:

• Act fast—the earlier you take action, the simpler this injury is to treat.

• Ice the area frequently, up to several times a day. Ice reduces inflammation and draws blood to the area to facilitate healing. Ice is one of the best self-treatments for healing tendinitis, but remember, this addresses only the damage already done; you must evaluate your shoes and training to avoid further trauma in the future. Do not ice immediately before running; allow an hour for the area to rewarm before exercise.

• Take an anti-inflammatory like aspirin or ibuprofen. As with ice, this can reduce pain and inflammation but will not solve the cause of your tendinitis.

• Stretch your calf area. Tightness in the calf is one of the causes of excess tugging on the Achilles tendon. Wait until the worst of the tendon trauma has subsided to begin a stretching regimen, so that you don't damage the tendon further. (See chapter 4 for lower leg stretches.)

• Examine your training and cut it back appropriately. Have you added hill workouts or speed workouts or both? Have you increased the duration of your long run? Tendinitis almost always occurs when training has been increased too fast in some manner. Cut back the workouts that you've added (and the ones that make your tendon the most sore afterward) and take your training down to a minimum while you're healing. A simple rule of thumb is that if your tendon is getting better with each day, your training is appropriate. If the pain is getting worse, you haven't cut your training enough.

• Evaluate your shoes. A major cause of tendinitis is shoes that do not give enough support. Consider buying a new model or adding a heel lift. Ask an educated staffer at a running shoe store or see a podiatrist to ensure that you are wearing appropriate shoes for your body type. Racing shoes often are a culprit. These flat shoes with not much of a heel can cause enough stress on the tendon to aggravate it in one race or training session.

• Consider physical therapy or massage if the above treatment does not resolve the problem.

• Surgery should generally be considered only if the tendon has actually ruptured to a severe degree.

Healing time. A week, if caught very early. Several weeks to a few months, if more advanced.

9

ALTERNATIVE TREATMENT CHOICES

GOING BEYOND CONVENTIONAL MEDICINE

Most runners visit a doctor or physical therapist when pain has made running uncomfortable or impossible—in other words, after they're hurt. But when it comes to injury prevention, a runner's best ally could be a practitioner of alternative medical therapy.

Alternative treatments—in particular, the practices of massage, acupuncture, and chiropractic medicine—have grown in popularity among athletes in general and runners specifically. These treatments are popular for their effectiveness at relaxing the body, reducing pain, and speeding recovery.

Professional athletes have been at the cutting edge of such therapies, long employing practitioners to ease their pains and prevent injury. Massage in particular is anything but "alternative" to professional runners—most elite runners consider a one-, two-, even three-times-a-week sports massage mandatory for their running health. Numerous other pro runners supplement their massage with visits to an acupuncturist or chiropractor. Serious runners consider these visits required maintenance for their very stressed bodies; they don't wait until they're hurt to seek treatment.

If the pros are putting their trust in these therapies, there's a good chance you can benefit, too. Here's a closer look at the most popular alternative treatments and how you can use them to get and stay healthy.

MASSAGE

Research has shown that massage can speed recovery and reduce muscle soreness associated with strenuous exercise. Massage also helps to maintain the muscles in their normal resting length. The more activity a muscle undergoes, the tighter it gets when idle, says Cynthia Ribeiro, a certified massage therapist, spokesperson for the American Massage Therapy Association, and owner of the Western Institute of Muscular Therapy in Laguna Hills, California. And if you don't counter the activity with relaxation, the muscle gets even tighter, she explains.

How it works. Massage (and sports massage in particular) increases bloodflow, realigns muscle fibers, and breaks up adhesions (scar tissue made up of collagen) that form during tissue healing. It also flushes toxins from the muscles—important for speeding your recovery—by stimulating and relaxing the system, explains Ribeiro, who has been training massage therapists and treating athletes for almost 20 years. "Blood brings oxygen to the muscles, and veins remove waste products," Ribeiro says. So if you encourage more ample bloodflow by relaxing the muscles, these pathways are freer to take away toxins. A relaxed muscle not only feels better than a tight muscle but is less likely to suffer strains and injury.

Many running injuries make themselves known slowly and only over time, and massage can identify potential problem spots. A good therapist will locate and work on minor aggravations—ones you didn't even know you had—before they become full-blown injuries. And because massage can speed healing and increase flexibility, it helps to neutralize some of the prime factors that lead to injury. In short, massage contributes to a runner's complete recovery.

If you're already injured, massage can still be a part of your treatment program. But don't get a massage in lieu of other treatment. Your massage therapist should work in conjunction with a team of appropriate sports medicine professionals.

In order to reap the full benefits of massage, visit a trained sports massage therapist. While Swedish or other conventional types of massage feel relaxing, these are generally not effective therapy for athletes. Sports massage is a deeper, more intense form of treatment than classic massage. Sports massage specialists are trained to target trigger points and adhesions. They know which muscles bear the brunt of particular sports and go after them aggressively.

As with all manner of practitioners, it's even better to find a therapist who specializes in treating runners—as opposed to athletes in general—since different sports take a toll on the body in unique ways.

What to expect. Advise your massage therapist of any pain or injury—both old and new. Most fresh injuries will likely require a lighter touch so as not to exacerbate swelling at the site. On the other hand, older injuries often call for stronger treatment, with cross-fiber friction—a rigorous, deep massaging of tissue intended to break up adhesions—where scarring has occurred. The therapist also will work on related tight or unbalanced areas that might have contributed to or resulted from the injury.

Sports massage can be uncomfortable but needn't be painful. The therapist must use a firm touch to be effective. However, you can and should communicate with your therapist if the pressure is too much for you. Together you can find a level of touch that feels right.

While runners' aches and pains tend to concentrate in the legs, most sports massage therapists will give a full-body massage, including the head, neck, shoulders, and arms. Welcome this attention, even if you came for a specific problem elsewhere. The therapist is not ignoring your crisis area but addressing other critical tension points. There's a good chance you have tender spots you didn't even know existed. (Some might have nothing to do with running but might be caused by other factors, such as sitting at a desk for hours on end.) Massaging the whole body enhances overall relaxation, a further step toward injury prevention.

Most massage therapists will ask you to undress to your level of comfort. While it's not necessary to remove underwear, there are points on the buttocks that are chronically tight on runners and that your masseuse might want to target.

The timing of massage is important. If you're not used to regular massage, an intense session can leave you feeling sluggish for a few days. If you want a full, deep massage before a race or hard workout and are accustomed to massage already, leave 3 days for recovery before the event. If you don't receive regular massages, leave 5 days to a week beforehand.

Gentle, stroking massage is safe right up until your hard effort, as well as immediately afterward. (Many marathons and large events have massage therapists on hand to administer postrace therapy.) Wait at least a day after your race to have deep tissue work. After a marathon, you'll want to wait even longer—up to a week if your muscle soreness is acute.

Regular maintenance massage is highly recommended for runners but can quickly get expensive. Many sports massage specialists advise runners to get on a program they can afford and that matches the intensity of their training. For example, if you're not training hard over the winter and running only easy distance, a massage once a month is fine. As you begin to gear up for racing in the spring, you might want a massage every other week. And if you are doing high mileage for a marathon and feeling particularly achy, it might be time to splurge for a month or two and get weekly massages.

How to find a practitioner. Choose a therapist specifically trained in sports massage and, better yet, one who specializes in treating runners. Because runners have running-specific injuries and tightness, this type of therapist will automatically know the spots to check and treat.

Begin by asking other runners and coaches in your area if they know of a good therapist. Check with your local running store, where practitioners might have brochures posted or the sales help might know of someone good. If you can't find a therapist in your area through word of mouth, visit www.amtamassage.org. Be sure to enter "sports specialty" into your search criteria.

ACUPUNCTURE

Acupuncture is an ancient form of Chinese medicine in which very thin needles are inserted into the body at specific points. The practice has grown in popularity in the West and is now available throughout the United States.

Acupuncture is used for myriad purposes, for everything from treating the common cold to providing anesthesia during surgery. And athletes have used it for centuries in China. "Throughout Chinese history, all the martial arts masters relied on acupuncture," says Yun-Tao Ma, Ph.D., a pain management specialist and doctor of Chinese medicine in Boulder, Colorado, who is at the forefront of studying and applying acupuncture treatment for athletes. "It was developed with sports in mind."

Today, the use of acupuncture in sports medicine is being rediscovered in the West. Unfortunately, Dr. Ma acknowledges, because there is little in the way of laboratory research on acupuncture, many athletes and medical doctors are not familiar with or convinced of its applications. But this is beginning to change, as research confirms and quantifies acupuncture's effects.

Perhaps the best thing about acupuncture is that it can never hurt. Some savvy runners use acupuncture before resorting to other invasive methods of treatment, including surgery, since acupuncture has no side effects or drawbacks. Other runners try acupuncture when everything else has failed—and wish they had turned to this form of medicine sooner.

How it works. According to traditional Chinese medicine experts, acupuncture works by helping to redirect the body's energy, or Qi. While that might sound a little fuzzy to Westerners, we can understand what's happening to a certain extent through more "scientific" language.

Acupuncture works on two levels. The process supplies oxygen and nutrients locally to individual muscles by stimulating and opening blood vessels. Systemically, or body-wide, it stimulates the nervous system to keep muscles, ligaments, and tendons working together. When a practitioner inserts the needles into the body's "motor" points (areas where nerves insert into muscle), it triggers the concentration of nerve bundles in the local area sending energy (Qi) through the meridians, or pathways, that are believed to run throughout the body. This in turn stimulates a homeostasis, or balance, within the nervous system. Without this balance, the joints cannot maintain good alignment, says Dr. Ma.

Acupuncture is a natural for preventing running injuries because the philosophy of traditional Chinese medicine addresses imbalances throughout the entire body, working to promote optimal health. In other words, a regular visit to the acupuncturist will identify and deal with problems before they develop into full-blown injuries. For example, a runner who is training hard and suffering from general fatigue and nonspecific pain is a great candidate for acupuncture. Because of the repetitive nature of running, muscles can develop tender, stressed areas prior to outright injury. "This will create pain, and the muscle will resist contraction," Dr. Ma says. Inserting needles into this stressed tissue restores proper function—both contraction and relaxation—of the muscle.

Acupuncture activates the healing process by stimulating nutrient and oxygen delivery to the muscles, according to experts in traditional Chinese medicine. In fact, studies have shown that acupuncture relieves

ACUPRESSURE POINTS FOR RUNNERS

A close cousin of acupuncture, acupressure is a treatment runners can perform on themselves. Acupressure relies on the same ancient system of meridians and points as acupuncture. The difference is that instead of inserting needles at these points, practitioners apply pressure with the hands, or sometimes the feet.

While the needle insertion of acupuncture is slightly more efficient, acupressure yields largely similar results, says Richard Gold, Ph.D., president of the International Professional School of Bodywork in San Diego, California.

For runners, acupressure is particularly effective for strains, spasms, and inflammation of muscle and connective tissue. It can be used to treat tenderness or as preventive maintenance. Runners who suffer from cramps, digestive difficulties, and "stitches" can also address those conditions with acupressure.

To self-treat with acupressure, follow these guidelines.

• Do it at a time when you are relaxed. Before or after a run is fine.

• Apply pressure with your fingers, thumbs, or heels firmly, but not to the point of pain, for 30 to 60 seconds.

• Breathe deeply during treatment.

• When possible, work the right- and left-side points at the same time. Otherwise, do one side first and then the other.

According to Dr. Gold, the following points are most helpful for runners.

pain, reduces inflammation, increases range of motion, and improves proprioception—how your body receives internal stimuli, crucial to understanding your body's location within space and therefore helpful to avoiding injury. In one study, acupuncture was used to treat shin splints, and the results were then compared with conventional physical therapy treatments. Subjects treated with just acupuncture recovered from exercise faster and had lower pain levels than those treated with physical therapy alone, according to Matthew Callison, a licensed acupuncturist,

POINT	LOCATION	BEST FOR
Urinary Bladder (UB) 36	Where the hamstring attaches to the buttocks (this point is best stimulated by the heels while kneeling)	Hamstring
UB 37	Directly in the middle of the hamstring (back of the thigh)	Hamstring
UB 40	Behind the knee	Hamstring, lower back
UB 57	Halfway up the center of the lower leg	Achilles tendon, calf, ankle
Gallbladder (GB) 31	Located where the middle finger touches the outside of the thigh while you're in a relaxed standing position	Sciatica, iliotibial ban
GB 34	Just below the knee on the outside of the leg	Connective tissue (ligaments and tendons), knee
Stomach (ST) 36	Just below GB 34	Gastrointestinal issues

certified athletic trainer, and owner of Acusport Life Center in San Diego, who conducted the research in conjunction with a team at the University of California, San Diego.

Acupuncture can address the root cause of certain running injuries; at the very least, it can alleviate accompanying pain. Many running injuries can be treated on several different levels, Callison says. For example, iliotibial (IT) band syndrome is caused by a muscle imbalance in the pelvis area, but runners experience the pain as friction in the knee.

Acupuncture treatment addresses IT band syndrome in three ways: It can help balance the pelvis, reduce strain on connective tissue caused by the restricted muscle, and reduce inflammation around the knee area.

As always, the runner must address the original cause of the injury for treatment to be fully successful. "Acupuncture will be a Band-Aid until any mechanical problems have been taken care of," Callison says. So if a runner has improper shoes or overpronates, those problems still must be solved. "Once that's taken care of, acupuncture will work better to balance the musculature and get rid of inflammation."

What to expect. Before your session begins, tell your practitioner of any pain or tightness you are experiencing. Be sure to mention any acute or chronic injury sites. Most practitioners will ask you to remove your clothes (except underwear) so they can target the necessary points. Needles can be inserted virtually anywhere on the body, from head to toe. Don't be surprised if your practitioner targets points in seemingly unrelated locations, as well as areas surrounding the discomfort.

Most practitioners use disposable needles, which vary in length up to several inches. (Choice of needle length depends on the depth of the point the practitioner is targeting and the muscle mass of the patient.) Despite the fearsome appearance of some acupuncture needles, there is little pain involved in the process. As the needle breaks the skin, expect to feel a stinging sensation that disappears almost immediately. A deeper twinge will follow as the practitioner inserts the needle to its proper depth, but this sensation also will dissipate quickly. In some cases, a sensation will travel from the site of the needle out toward an extremity. This "referral" is a good thing, suggesting a target has been hit solidly.

You should never feel shooting or stabbing pain—if you do, mention it to your acupuncturist, who will likely remove and replace the offending needle. Some people will experience minor soreness after a session of acupuncture. This is considered normal but should disappear within 24 hours.

If your goal is to prevent injury and improve performance, expect to visit the acupuncturist once a week or every other week. This can vary depending on the practitioner, your state of health, and your budget. You can receive a treatment the day before a hard workout or a race, but be sure to inform your practitioner so that he can adjust the technique accordingly.

For injury treatment, the duration and frequency of your visits will depend on the severity and nature of your injury, and the practitioner. Acute injuries generally require fewer treatments than chronic injuries (except in the case of massive tears that require long healing periods). For ongoing or old injuries, most practitioners will want to see patients once or twice a week for several weeks.

If you can't afford a long-term program of treatment, don't write off acupuncture entirely. Just one session can help alleviate the pain and inflammation of an acute injury. And most practitioners will be happy to work with you to find a program of treatment that will be both effective and affordable.

How to find a practitioner. Look for one specifically trained in treating athletes and, better yet, one who focuses on runners. Word of mouth is the best way to do so. Inquire whether other local runners use an acupuncturist; your local running store is a good place to ask. If there is a sports medicine clinic in your area, the staff there might be able to direct you to a good practitioner. Callison welcomes visitors to his Web site, www.acusporthealth.com, from which he can help locate a local practitioner.

CHIROPRACTIC

Chiropractic treatment is a hands-on therapy approach that focuses on the manipulation of joints. It is noninvasive and does not involve any drugs or surgery, instead relying on mechanical movement of the body to restore proper function.

As with acupuncture, chiropractic focuses on injury and disease prevention. Practitioners take a holistic approach, viewing and treating the whole body.

An ongoing relationship with a practitioner who knows your body and training could prove beneficial in preventing injury. "A chiropractor might be able to locate a restriction that the runner might not be aware of," says Boston-based chiropractor Margaret Karg, a former president of the American Chiropractic Association's Council on Sports Injuries and Physical Fitness. Many runners see chiropractors on a regular basis, using the treatment as one would tune up a car to ensure that all systems are functioning properly.

Chiropractors treat a wide variety of running injuries. Back pain often draws an athlete to a practitioner initially, but treatment isn't limited to back problems. From ankle sprains to iliotibial band syndrome, chiropractic can relieve pain and work to restore normal functioning.

If you establish a relationship with a chiropractic practice and the treatments work for you, consider making it your first stop when you are suffering pain or injury. With their training, chiropractors should be able to determine if you need to visit a medical doctor. And your practitioner should be willing to work as part of a team of treatment that will depend on the injury.

How it works. By manipulating the body, a chiropractor seeks to correct a restriction of proper joint play. When a joint is "cavitated," eliciting the familiar cracking sound, the glide of the joint is improved and often with it the range of motion. Both of these can in turn reduce pain.

While the stereotypical image of a chiropractor draws up images of spinal manipulation, in fact chiropractors look at and treat the whole body, says Dr. Karg. In addition, chiropractors will also prescribe reha-

WHAT THE PROS KNOW

WHY TO START A TREATMENT HABIT

A busy lifestyle can make scheduling a visit to the massage therapist or acupuncturist easily forgotten. And with finances tight for many of us, it can be hard to justify treatment until you're actually in pain. But in the case of all these alternative treatments, a little bit of time and money spent on maintenance can prevent much larger bills and time commitments spent treating a serious injury.

To ensure that you're taking proper care of yourself, build regular appointments into your calendar during times of intense training. This is especially important when you're coming back from injury, preparing for a marathon, or gearing up for race season. Schedule several visits months ahead of time, so that you know you won't be shut out during a busy time or be surprised when your practitioner is out of town.

bilitation therapy and even nutritional advice, depending on the health issues of the patient.

What to expect At your first visit, expect a thorough consultation in which you discuss your general health history and any specific issues. Your chiropractor will then conduct a physical examination, including general tests such as blood pressure and reflexes, and specific orthopedic tests to determine range of motion and functioning of various body parts. In some cases, your practitioner may request more extensive diagnostic exams. (Many chiropractors can take x-rays in their office, and they might refer you elsewhere for other tests, including MRIs.)

Treatment might begin on the first visit, if the chiropractor has sufficient time and information. The practitioner will manipulate and adjust key joints. He might also use physical therapy modalities, such as ultrasound or electrical stimulation. Depending on the patient's situation, the chiropractor might also prescribe exercises to improve strength or flexibility.

Chiropractic manipulation, the hands-on part of the treatment, should not be painful. Some patients will experience general muscle soreness the next day, but this should dissipate rapidly. The less conditioned an athlete, the more likely he or she is to feel this temporary discomfort.

Treatment will vary depending on the nature of the injury and the severity of the pain. In some cases, one treatment might do the trick. In the case of more challenging or chronic injury, a practitioner might want to see you frequently—once or twice a week—during actual treatment and then less often for follow-up visits.

For general preventive maintenance, as with massage and acupuncture, your program of treatment will depend on your practitioner, your overall health, and your budget. Work with your chiropractor to determine a course of action that will be most beneficial to you.

Unlike other treatments, chiropractic can be performed immediately before an athletic event. In fact, some professional athletes plan their visits for before races, believing they will have optimal functioning and range of motion if they've been treated just prior to strenuous activity.

However, don't go for your first-ever visit to a chiropractor right before your big race. In order to see how your body reacts, familiarize yourself with the treatment and your practitioner with several visits in the weeks leading up to your event.

If you are experiencing pain after a race, Dr. Karg recommends waiting a day before seeing a chiropractor. Pain might abate and sensations change and settle. If pain persists after 24 hours, a visit to a chiropractor is definitely in order.

How to find a practitioner. Chiropractors are considered primary health-care practitioners, so you won't need a referral from your medical doctor. Look for a chiropractor certified in one of the two sports categories: They'll have the letters CCSP (Certified Chiropractic Sports Physician) or DACBSP (Diplomate American Chiropractic Board of Sports Physicians) after their name. Many sports medicine clinics have chiropractors who specialize in recreational athletics.

To locate a chiropractor in your area, visit www.amerchiro.org. You can search the database by location and sports certification. Another good resource is www.chirodirectory.com.

10

ATTITUDE IS EVERYTHING

THE EMOTIONAL SIDE OF INJURY

Your attitude can prevent an injury. Sound farfetched? It's not. Runners who are obsessed with their workouts sometimes are not willing to take time off when the early warning signs of an injury present themselves. This inability to take a break—even just 1 day off—can mean the difference between a mild aggravation and a full-blown injury.

WHEN RUNNING BECOMES AN OBSESSION

You might know runners who place too much importance on their running. They're the ones limping through their workouts, a chronic litany of aches and pains spilling from their lips. Yet they continue running without a break. They continue racing. They schedule their work and family life—even vacations—around their runs instead of the other way around.

The percentage of runners for whom running is a true behavioral addiction is fairly small, according to sports psychologists. In fact, experts generally don't apply the term "addiction" to such behaviors as running or gambling the way they do to substance dependencies such as alcohol or tobacco. Nevertheless, whether you choose to call them addicted, obsessive, compulsive, or just out of control, some runners just don't know when it's time to stop.

Runners who are obsessive lose the ability to make choices. Logging their daily miles is not up for debate, no matter the weather, other commitments, or the way they feel physically. Faced with mounting deadlines at work, say, or flitting pain in their legs, addicted runners won't consider taking the day off. They are extremely rigid about sticking to the schedule or plan. If the goal was 50 miles for the week, nothing less will satisfy. And if they've targeted a race in a few weeks, they'll keep their sights on that race, even when training results and other body signs indicate they might not be ready at all; that they are, in fact, about to hurt themselves badly.

These runners feel listless and grumpy when something finally does force them to take a break. Nothing else will do—forget swimming and biking, which don't provide the same euphoria—and they don't feel quite themselves until they can get back to their "daily fix."

Of course, many runners—even very committed ones—have no problem taking a few days off. These are the runners who, faced with deadlines at work or a sore hamstring, figure, "Today's a good day to take off and rest." Instead of addiction, their running is a healthy habit. They still have control over their choice to run.

RECOGNIZING A PROBLEM

It's quite normal for you to feel down when you can't do your usual workout. Your body becomes accustomed to regular aerobic exercise, and physiological changes when you suddenly stop—including sleep, appetite, intestinal, and mood disruptions—are not just imagined. But it's one thing to be a little bummed out and quite another to be outright flattened.

The difference between a runner who's dedicated and one who's obsessed is in how well they function when *not* running, says Deborah Greenslit, a sports psychologist at the Center for Psychological Skills Training for Coaches and Athletes in Paxton, Massachusetts, who's run 30 marathons of her own. Addicted runners tend to be very stressed and exhausted, says Jane Welzel, a psychotherapist specializing in sports psychology in Fort Collins, Colorado, and a marathoner who competed for years at an elite level.

For these people, it's not the running that's at fault. Rather the obsession is largely the result of the runner's personality. "If you're predisposed to addiction in general, then you're more prone to become addicted to running," Greenslit says. And if the addiction weren't running, chances are it would be cycling or shopping or something else.

Your chances of becoming obsessed boil down to the strength of

WHAT THE PROS KNOW

SHORT-TERM GAIN = LONG-TERM PAIN

Runners who make a living in the sport must be adept at keeping their long-term interests in mind. If they ignore a small pain that then flares into a weeks-long injury, they can be out of contention for an entire competitive season. It's no exaggeration that oftentimes it's not the fastest runner who wins a race but the one who trains the smartest to avoid injuries. If your short-term training plan doesn't help further your ultimate goals, then you need to make adjustments.

To benefit from a similar, long-term outlook, ask yourself the questions that Jane Welzel, a psychotherapist specializing in sports psychology in Fort Collins, Colorado, asks her clients.

• What is your overall running goal?

• What is the purpose of today's run?

• Does today's run put you closer to or farther from that long-term goal?

Say your big goal race is a marathon 2 months away and you plan to run a half-marathon this coming weekend as a tough training run for the marathon. But yesterday you felt a strain growing in your tendon during your track workout. The answers to these questions will show you that running the half-marathon on a sore tendon could set you back from your larger goal—you'll likely wind up with a severe strain that takes weeks of rest to heal. The more difficult, but much smarter, decision that better suits your long-term goals would be to cancel this weekend's race plans, take a few days of rest and recovery, and resume your training when you feel better.

your coping mechanisms, Welzel says. How well are you able to tolerate changes in your emotional state? People who possess the internal resources to comfort and calm themselves in times of crisis are less likely to use running, or anything else, as an emotional crutch.

How can you tell if you're addicted? Ask yourself these questions: Do you feel agitated and anxious when you can't run? Do you trust that you have the discipline to get back on board when you are able to resume? "When runners are addicted," says Greenslit, "it feeds an irritability when they can't run, and you won't see any flexibility."

WHAT'S SO BAD ABOUT BEING OBSESSED?

Since running is a "positive" obsession (exercise is good for you!), it's natural to wonder why it would be a problem. It's not hurting anyone . . . or is it?

"An obsessed runner is more likely to suffer injury," Greenslit says. Because these runners are motivated largely by the obsession, rather than their goals, they'll run through injuries despite the pain and the risk of further injury.

Here's what happens. Most running injuries start small and present themselves gradually. A nonaddicted runner can head off most injuries during this time simply by paying attention to signs and listening to his body. But the addicted runner is incapable of such logical action. He ignores those first warnings. In fact, he ignores all the warnings. Then, inevitably, he gets hurt. "These runners are unwilling, unable, or afraid to take even a day off," explains Welzel.

In a way, it's amazing that someone could love something so much that it results in utterly counterproductive behavior. But that's what addicted runners do. They run themselves right into the ground, often ending up with such severe injuries that they are forced to take a long layoff.

If you're obsessive about your running (and even if you're not), consider these strategies for nurturing a healthier attitude.

Learn the difference between injury and normal discomfort. Running through injury is not the same as running through minor discomfort. Running on an injury virtually always makes it more severe and prolongs the healing process. A minor tendon aggravation that you run

WHEN TO GET HELP

If you think your running might be out of control, start with some self-therapy, says Michael Sachs, Ph.D., a specialist in sports psychology and a professor of kinesiology at Temple University in Philadelphia. Read up on exercise addiction and try taking action on your own. "Ask yourself what would be involved in pulling back, take stock of your running, try some other activities," he says. Give yourself a season, or several months, of running to see if you can make progress. "Then if that doesn't work, seeing a sports psychologist is a good idea."

on repeatedly can lead to a ruptured tendon. A minor case of runner's knee can rub and scrape until you need surgery to run comfortably. Running under such circumstances is counterproductive.

The tricky thing here is that training involves stressing your system in order to strengthen it. Progress, therefore, necessitates a certain amount of discomfort. If we stopped running at the first sign of pain, we'd never become runners.

So, when does tough become just plain stupid? That's the question runners struggle with constantly. A few lucky runners are gifted with a strong sense of what their bodies can handle—they know when to push through general discomfort but also recognize when pain is out of the ordinary and must be heeded. For most runners, this sensibility comes only with maturity and trial and error. Most of us learn the hard way (which is to say, by suffering injuries) that time off to halt an injury is not wimping out but playing it smart. A rule of thumb to start with is that general muscle soreness—for example, legs that are tired and a bit achy from yesterday's hilly run—is acceptable. Any pain involving joints or connective tissue is an immediate red flag, as is muscle soreness specific to one location, indicating a strain or pull.

Have patience. Welzel learned all about patience after suffering a broken neck in a car accident while training in New Zealand. She almost lost her life, and throughout her recovery, she was told running would no longer be realistic. "I was forced to take time off—there was not a lot I could do," she says. "I had to have a lot of patience. I learned through that process that if I rushed, I always set myself back. There are no shortcuts. You'll end up compensating with some other injury." Her lesson was severe, but she says she learned infinite patience that she's called upon for the rest of her running career (which, as it turns out, has been a long and successful one).

Remember who else you are. For dedicated runners, the sport is not only how we spend our time, it becomes who we are. Our friends are runners, we plan and eat meals that benefit our running, we spend our spare time reading about running. These are healthy aspects of a hobby that fills a large part of our lives.

But obsessed runners feel lost without this identity. These runners don't know how to "be" if their day doesn't revolve around running. Faced with this deep absence, they continue to run even when it is counterproductive. A slow run, even a painful run, is better than no run to the addicted runner who relies solely on this athletic sense of self.

That's why it's important to remember your "other" identities. Are you a father, mother, artist, lawyer, husband, wife? More than one of these? You will still be a runner even if you don't run every day. Don't let your running identity fuel your running; leave that to your other identity—you will be a much stronger mother or father or lawyer if you don't get hurt.

Give yourself choices. This is the most elemental separation between the healthy runner and the compulsive one. The addicted runner never allows himself the option of not running—it just doesn't exist. He is no longer in control of his running; instead, it controls him. In the absence of the ability to make choices, the runner continues to run even when all signs are pointing toward injury. But you do have choices. Find another activity—swimming, yoga, Pilates—and put your runner's mentality to work mastering it. You'll achieve a sense of accomplishment along with the fitness benefits. (See chapters 5 and 6 for more on strength training and cross-training.)

So what's so bad about being obsessed? Plenty, it turns out. There's the very real heightened risk of injury. And there's also the toll on the rest of the runner's life. After all, all the energy that goes into running has to come from somewhere.

"If people get obsessed about anything, they lose their balance in their life," Welzel says. "Other things suffer, like relationships or jobs. If they have to run no matter what, they'll miss the kid's ballgame or not go to an important function.

"Also, they get just stressed out, because life is making it hard for them to get their run in. Their days become longer, and they don't get enough rest, because there's just no option not to do it."

Greenslit, who finally gained a healthier perspective after her own injuries forced her to curtail her obsessive running, says there's nothing healthy about a running obsession. "It was driving me—you can exhaust yourself literally, running twice a day. It was not necessarily a healthy perspective." She changed, she says, when she realized, "It was more important for me to be able to run for the rest of my life than to run every day of my life."

THE INJURY-DEPRESSION CONNECTION

We've seen how your emotional state can hurt you. But once injured, runners have different emotional issues to deal with. Treating an injury is not as simple as icing it and taking a few days off. The anxiety and depression it brings on are sometimes as debilitating as the physical damage. That's not just for addicted runners. Any dedicated runner can suffer the blues when sidelined.

"It's natural to feel down when you're injured," Welzel says. "Running becomes a way of life, so you miss the routine, the camaraderie, how it makes you feel." And not being able to run because you're injured can make you feel out of control, especially if it's an injury you don't understand or know how to treat.

That loss of control is a prime cause of depression during a forced layoff. We runners are a control-hungry group. We measure our miles and times, weeks and months so carefully. We plan our training months, even years, in advance. So an injury that deflates this sense of control is hard to take.

Other factors conspire to bring on the blahs as well, in particular the loss of fitness—real or perceived—that you've worked so hard to gain and the general malaise brought on by suddenly ceasing physical activity. The end result might not be true clinical depression but a perfectly valid down-in-the-dumps feeling. It's a normal response, Greenslit explains.

THE POWER OF POSITIVE

I defy you to find a successful professional runner with a downbeat attitude. A huge part of running well is due to believing in yourself, and if you fall prey to feeling sorry for yourself, you'll never be able to run to your full potential.

That attitude is critical not just in racing and training but perhaps even more so in handling setbacks. In some cases, it's what separates the champions from the also-rans. Facing injury with assurance and a fiercely bright outlook will help you get the right care for your injury, do everything possible to speed healing, and return to training with intelligence and patience.

What the pros know is how to stay positive. They surround themselves with positive people—coaches and other runners who look on the bright side as well, who seek the lessons from all experiences, bad or good. Talk to doctors, coaches, other runners. Read up on your injury. Look forward to your comeback. Your injury might have taken control of your training temporarily, but you still have control of your life and your outlook.

Normal, yes. Fun? No way. Any runner who's experienced the interruption an injury brings to his routine is familiar with the frustration, the anger, the sadness. But it's what you do with those emotions that is important. Moping around won't help the injury heal any faster and can make the situation feel worse than it really is. Focusing intently on the negative—in any situation, not just running injuries—is a recipe for unhappiness.

A running injury can result in outright depression, but only in a small percentage of cases, and usually results from a layoff of several weeks or more—or a career-ending injury. How do you know if you've crossed the line? "When it begins to interfere with your everyday functioning, then it becomes a concern," Greenslit says. "What's not okay is when you can't get out of bed."

LOOK ON THE BRIGHT SIDE

It sounds cliché enough to ignore. And it *is* tough to look on the bright side when you need to take off 2 weeks to heal a muscle pull or 6 weeks to mend a stress fracture. But it's more than just a silly saying. Focusing on the positive during your injury can help you heal faster and feel better. Here are a few things to try the next time you're sidelined.

Find the lesson. As we saw earlier in this book, most running injuries happen for a reason. They are overuse injuries set in motion by rapid training changes, improper shoes, sudden changes in terrain, or any of a dozen such factors.

Once you're injured, play detective and attempt to learn where you went wrong. Analyze your training (and the results of it) for clues. Did you suddenly start training on a hilly trail several times a week? Did you fail to replace your favorite shoes, even after wearing them for 6 months? Did you not heed early warning signs like an ache deep in your muscle or tendon soreness that grew worse by the day?

Talk to other runners about their experiences with similar injuries and read up on the issue in books and on Web sites. What can you learn about your training? Your personality? Your outlook on running and on life? By focusing on learning—rather than just berating yourself for making mistakes—you are taking control. And any time you take control, you reduce your feelings of depression. The big bonus: You're also less likely to make the same mistake again.

Focus on the future. Allow yourself a day or two of sulking, then move on. After that, it's counterproductive. There's no going back in time, and it doesn't do any good to kick yourself for mistakes you made that led to your injury. Negativity feeds depression and feelings of hopelessness.

Instead, spend your downtime mapping out a realistic future training plan that gradually brings you back to fitness. Make adjustments based on what you've learned about your training by analyzing your previous injuries and performance. Set goals that include a reasonable starting point and a very gradual return to fitness. Creating a plan will give you some control over your recovery process.

Manage your injury. It's maddening to sit there and wait while your body takes its own sweet time to heal. That's why it helps to know that you are doing everything you can to speed the process of healing. Make sure you've seen the proper medical practitioners. Get answers to all your questions. Follow up your doctor visits with a trip to a physical therapist and ask for a rehabilitation program you can work on at home. Use your extra time to make other changes that will help your training next time around: Does your diet need adjusting with extra protein or calcium? Could you be doing a more comprehensive stretching routine? By being an active manager of your injury, you minimize feelings of loss and helplessness.

Cross-train. I know, I know—nothing can match running. Swimming and cycling just aren't the same. Yoga and weight lifting don't get you out of breath. Nothing gives you the same buzz as your favorite sport. Still, something is better than nothing. Cross-training will help you maintain at least some of your hard-earned fitness.

Look for activities that stress both your cardiovascular and your muscular systems. And of course, don't do anything that exacerbates your injury. (For more on good cross-training activities for various injuries, see chapter 6.)

There's a side benefit to cross-training, too: While you focus on staying in shape during your layoff, the physical activity is generating endorphins that boost your mood.

Do something entirely different. Forget training altogether and relish your temporary bonanza of extra time. That hour a day you filled with running is prime time to spend on hobbies or family commitments that have been taking a back seat. Whip the garden into shape. Read a good book. Take the children to the zoo. Allow yourself to remember all the things you don't even consider when you're too busy running.

Instead of looking at your injury as a horrible break in your life when time stops, view this as a gift of time. Spend it how you like and treasure the moments, rather than counting days until they're over. I'll admit—this recommendation becomes easier as your running career matures. If you're deep in the heart of competition, it's hard to find happiness in weeding the garden. But after you've been through a few injuries and you understand that they are a normal part of the running cycle, it's easier to relax and enjoy your breaks and use the time productively.

Use positive imagery and self-talk. These psychological skills can help to reduce feelings of anxiety and maintain a positive outlook. Picture your injury healing properly and fast. Envision yourself running

WHAT YOU CAN DO

Analyze your attitude. Are you in control of your running or does it control you? Do you feel you must run every day, even when you are feeling sick or have other pressing commitments?

Remember your nonrunning identity. If you feel you are running obsessively to the exclusion of other parts of your life, consider a session with a sports psychologist. You can gain insights into other subjects of interest, such as performance and competition.

Think positive. Enough said.

Find other outlets for your energy. Focus on other favorite pursuits (fitness-related or not) that you don't have time for when you are running.

Learn from experience. Always analyze your training. What sudden changes did you make in training? Were you wearing worn-out shoes? Figure out what you'll do differently next time around.

strong once again. Set aside a few minutes each day for these visualizations, or do it whenever you find yourself stressing about your injury.

Likewise, positive self-talk can nip feelings of depression in the bud. "Instead of saying 'Woe is me,' ask 'How can I use this to my advantage?'" says Michael Sachs, Ph.D., a specialist in sports psychology and a professor of kinesiology at Temple University in Philadelphia. "Tell yourself you're going to run smart when you come back."

Remember, it could be worse. Find a positive whenever you are drawn toward the negative. For example, if you can jog for only 1 mile, remind yourself that just 2 weeks ago you couldn't run at all. Sometimes, the positive aspect is that the injury might be a blessing in disguise: Maybe the forced layoff saved you from overtraining, which would have led to complications of its own. Sometimes, dedicated runners don't take enough voluntary training breaks, and injury is the only break they get. In this case, your break might save you from a compromised immune system, leaden-feeling legs, and a frustrating plateau in training. You'll feel refreshed once you return to running and will be better able to train in the long run.

Let it go. Most of these techniques focus on regaining control in order to reduce feelings of loss and helplessness. But there's a flip side to all that. Once you've done everything you can to be sure you're on the path back to health, let it go. Don't spend the whole day obsessing about your injury. Do what you can and recognize when you can't do anymore. Focus your attention elsewhere when it's not doing any active good. Just fretting is not time well-spent and certainly won't help the healing process.

IT'S ALL ABOUT PERSPECTIVE

All these suggestions have something in common: They are all ways you can create something positive from your injury. And that's one thing you truly control—your outlook during your injury is entirely up to you. Once the physical damage of an injury is done, there's no going back. There's only the opportunity to make the experience as good as possible, rather than a dismal time to suffer through.

Running injuries are not the end of the world (although sometimes they seem like it). So keep things in perspective. There's always another summer. Always another race to train for. Yes, you've worked hard. Yes, you're suffering a setback. But in the grand scheme of your life, is this really something to fret over? Odds are good that you'll be able to resume your favorite sport soon enough.

11

A NEW RUNNER'S SAFETY PRIMER

START SLOW, STAY WELL

The hardest part about running is starting. Your body isn't used to the motion, the stresses, the pounding. It all feels strange and uncomfortable. It does get easier with time, but your first weeks and months as a runner are critical because your unconditioned body is more susceptible to injury.

"People make the mistake of playing their sports to get in shape—and not getting in shape to play their sports," says John Cavanaugh, a physical therapist at Women's Sports Medicine Center at the Hospital for Special Surgery in New York City who specializes in treating runners and has worked with the New York City Marathon. Runners especially need to take this into consideration to avoid injury.

That means you must start gradually and build your training incrementally. You also need to supplement your running with other strength and cardiovascular activities early on, until you're fit enough to handle more running.

As you learn to heed your body's messages with greater wisdom and your body grows acclimated to the repetitive motion of running, injury becomes less likely. Here's some guidance to take you from those early stages of the sport and give you the chance to become a cagey veteran.

STARTING OFF ON THE RIGHT FOOT

Running tends to get a terrible rap from newcomers. But it's not the running that's so awful. It's the manner in which new runners begin to train.

Beginners typically run too hard, too fast, and too long on their first few attempts. To top it off, they wear the wrong shoes, ones that give them little support and not enough cushioning. So you've got a sudden shock to the body with little to no protection from the one piece of equipment required for running. It's no surprise that these are the folks who say, "I hate running! I tried it, and it hurt too much."

The experience tends to be not only extremely uncomfortable but also a terrific way to get injured before really getting started. Aching knees, tender Achilles tendons, and sore shins have stopped plenty of new runners in their tracks.

Pain should never be part of the normal running experience. Sure, discomfort is to be expected as your body adjusts and your muscles get stronger. But agony shouldn't be a given in running.

So why do so many people experience these painful false starts in running? Because most of them believe they can jump into this sport without any guidance. Running seems simple. But it's deceptively so. People think, "Heck, anyone can run. Running is child's play, something we do naturally since the age of 2. No special skills must be learned, no instruction involved, no difficult equipment mastered."

In fact, turning yourself into a runner is a tough proposition. It takes smarts and guidance to evolve gradually enough to keep stepping up to the next level. It takes patience to gain the strength and endurance that will allow you to continue your running program. As a beginner, you'll be served better by an open mind and a student's perspective than any tough-it-out attitude.

Learning about how the body adapts to the stresses of running is your most important first step, so you're on the right path by reading this book. An extremely gradual buildup is the key to getting started, as are a few precautionary measures. Here's a plan for running healthy and injury-free.

Get a health check. You've heard it before, but it's worth repeating—and heeding. Seeing a physician for an overall examination is a good idea, particularly if you're at risk for heart disease, which is the primary reason those health checks are advised any time someone starts a new exercise program. That means a health exam is essential if you are overweight, if your family has a history of high cholesterol, high blood pressure, or heart disease; or if you have any of those symptoms yourself.

Even if your family health history and your own are impeccable, it's not a bad idea to get checked out before you start a running program. Your physician might discover other hidden disease that would impact your health and training. Osteoporosis and anemia, for example, commonly go undetected in women.

By checking in with a doctor, you'll find out if you need to be monitored closely as you proceed with your exercise or if you must be treated for any conditions that could be affected by your exercise routine. Beginning a running program without addressing such problems can exacerbate them and possibly lead to injury or more severe health complications.

Get the right shoes for your body type. The first pair of running shoes you buy is the most important pair you'll choose. That's because if you're in the wrong shoes, everything from your feet up to your knees, hips, and back could wind up hurting. Too many runners have been turned off to the sport because of wearing improper shoes.

Beginners might not understand the concept of the body as a series of links in a chain. Your feet, as the point of impact with the ground, are the most critical link in this series of connections that your body comprises. That means that foot problems that are not addressed can end up hurting higher up in the chain: ankles, knees, hips, and back. A new runner whose knees hurt typically will think the problem is that he "just isn't cut out for running." What this runner doesn't realize is that a simple shoe change will reduce torque on his knees and align his legs and feet properly. Suddenly, he *is* cut out for running.

It may not always work that simply, but shoes are the most important place to start on your path to comfortable, injury-free running. So *don't* go for your first run in any old tennis shoes you have moldering in the closet. And don't, if you can help it, go to a generic department store and choose a pair of running shoes that just look good to you. Shop at a running specialty store—one that's staffed by runners for runners. These stores stake their livelihood on the fact that their staff can help you match the right shoe with your unique foot and stride.

Once you're a more experienced runner, you'll become familiar with the way your feet and legs are "supposed" to feel and the way in which different shoes help or hurt your foot placement and therefore make you feel better or worse. At that point, you'll be better able to make your own choices in shoes—although it's still a good idea to patronize a running store if one is available in your area, since they'll have the largest selection and the most informed sales staff.

What are the best shoes for you? The ones that feel good, minimize your chance of injury, and serve your running purpose well. Here are a few ground rules for beginners.

• **Brand name doesn't matter.** Brand *fit* does. Every major running shoe manufacturer makes perfectly good shoes. That means that brand preference comes down largely to the matter of fit: Each brand builds its shoes on a different last, or shoe shape. So some will be wider in the heel, others in the toe box, and so forth. Invariably, one brand or another will conform to the outline of your foot more naturally than others. That's the brand you want to go with. Nike and Asics, for example, are known for fitting narrow feet better. Saucony and Adidas are known for wider toe boxes. Also, New Balance has always offered shoes in variable widths, and now other manufacturers are doing so as well. Most of the major running shoe manufacturers design men's and women's shoes on gender-specific lasts. The women's shoes typically have narrower heels and a longer, slimmer toe box than men's. A few women with wide feet do prefer men's models, but most feel more comfortable in women's shoes.

• **Your best friend's favorite shoe doesn't matter.** Running shoes are built with different body and foot types in mind. So the shoe your friend swears by might in fact be disastrous for you. It might allow your foot to roll in too much and strain your ankles, or it might not provide enough cushioning. Choosing a shoe means finding the one that's right for your own individual running stride.

• **Spend a little money.** Once you see the selection of shoes in the store, you'll surely wonder why you should fork over $135 for a pair of shoes when some are only $50. In fact, you don't have to go with the top of the line, but do plan to spend at least $70 or $80. That's because those few extra dollars buy you the technology that goes into making the shoe specifically constructed for running and for you. Bottom-of-the-line running shoes, for the most part, do not contain the components designed to cushion and control abnormalities in the running stride—they are essentially athletic shoes without running-specific features. The more expensive shoes are designed to help even out your stride and minimize your biomechanical problems, therefore protecting you from injury. You don't need to buy the most expensive pair in the store, but to get a viable training shoe, you'll at least want to get something in the mid-price range or higher. The cheapest shoes, quite simply, are more for walking around than for running. (For more specifics on footwear and how to know which type of shoe is best for you, see chapter 3.)

Walk and run when you first get started. Running places greater stresses on your body than walking does. For a new runner, that means that joints, muscles, tendons, ligaments, and even bones all must be conditioned to those stresses to avoid discomfort, not to mention strains, tears, and other injury. As we established earlier in this chapter, doing too much too soon is a significant cause of injury among newcomers, since the conditioning of soft tissues and bones can lag behind the body's cardiovascular ability.

The best way to slowly indoctrinate your body to running is to alternate periods of walking and jogging. These intervals can start out very short for people who have not been doing any regular exercise: jogging for 15 to 20 seconds and then walking an equal period of time. If you're more fit aerobically, alternate 1 minute of jogging with 1 minute of walking for your starting point.

After several days of this, lengthen the intervals. If you've been alternating periods of 20 seconds, increase those to 30 seconds, then after a few more days to 45 seconds. Eventually, when you have increased to 2 minutes of jogging, you can shorten your walking breaks so that you are running more than you are walking. Start alternating 2 minutes of jogging with 1 minute of walking. Then 3 minutes of jogging with 1 minute of walking. When you get up to 5 minutes, you can start to phase out the walking altogether. Do longer stretches of jogging with just a brief walking break. For example, jogging 10 minutes, walking 1 minute, and jogging 10 minutes again.

Your overall goal as a beginner should be to eventually jog for 30 minutes straight without walking. This goal can take anywhere from a few days to a few months to achieve, depending on your initial fitness level. Follow your own schedule and don't rush; it's better to be consistent and progress gradually than to start off like gangbusters and have to stop after a few days or weeks. Conditioning occurs gradually in the body, and there's no way to hurry the process. Even if you are *aerobically* fit and able to jog a few miles at a stretch right away, your body still has to adapt to the impact of running.

Run slower than you think you should. Your goal as a beginner should not be to run as fast as you can. It should be to gradually increase the length of time you are able to run until you can comfortably jog for about half an hour. Only after you reach this milestone should you even think about your pace.

Speed comes with time and conditioning. Your musculature must develop strength to propel you more efficiently so you can run faster. This will happen naturally, and eventually you can do more speed-specific workouts. But for a beginner, *completion* is the goal, not minutes per mile.

One of the most basic rules of training and injury prevention is that a runner should not increase both distance and intensity at the same time. So it follows logically that if you're a beginner, focusing all your energy on covering the distance by jogging instead of walking, you shouldn't even think about intensity (speed) until you can comfortably cover your goal distance.

By focusing on a gradual increase in the duration of your runs, you allow all the systems in your body to get used to running a little at a time. Your bones and muscles will get stronger; tendons and ligaments will become used to the massive forces generated when running. You are ensuring that the load placed on your body is growing incrementally, minimizing the chance of injury.

Don't run every day. Rest days are crucial for repair and rejuvenation of all parts of your body. Work without rest is a recipe for breakdown and injury.

Beginning runners should aim to run 3 or 4 days a week. Alternate 2 days of running/walking with a rest day. Don't go too far in the other direction, though. If you run only every third day or so, that won't be frequent enough to see any improvement.

The 2 days on, 1 day off schedule is just right for beginners to gain conditioning without overstressing their bodies. After a month or so of this schedule, increase to 3 or 4 days of running, then take a day off.

Most runners will benefit from taking off 1 day a week, even when highly conditioned. The chances of injury increase for runners who never take a day off, and injury incidence has been directly tied to the number of consecutive days that athletes run. A rest day allows microtears to heal and inflammation to subside. It's like having an insurance policy for your body to protect yourself against injuries you don't even have yet. For all but professional runners, 1 day a week should always be taken off for rest and recuperation.

Cross-train to increase fitness. While you shouldn't run every day as a beginner, you can and should do other exercise that complements running. This will help you to get in shape, build muscles that running doesn't emphasize, and minimize the chances of injury.

Cross-training is more helpful for new runners than experienced runners, says physical therapist Cavanaugh. Veteran runners' bodies are able to withstand the stresses of running on a daily basis. Beginners can't run that much, so they need to build their heart and lungs and burn calories in other ways. Activities such as swimming, biking, lifting weights, and using an elliptical trainer all help newcomers to get in shape without the joint pounding of running.

Do one or two cross-training activities on your days off from running. (For more on cross-training, see chapter 6.)

Listen to your body. One of the hardest things for new runners to ascertain is just how they should be feeling when they are running. You're out of breath, your heart is racing. Everything feels weird. Every-

LISTEN CAREFULLY

Runners and other endurance athletes who really learn to listen to their bodies sometimes are even able to sense nonrunning-related illness early on, since they are tipped off to early warning signals by a perceptible drop in running ability. Many veteran runners have picked up on evidence of thyroid disease, immune system disorders, even cancer due to noticeable changes in their training. Chances are sedentary people wouldn't have noticed symptoms until they became more dramatic. In this way, running performance can serve as a general barometer of health and wellness for those who are truly in tune with their bodies.

thing feels sore. "Everyone says 'Listen to your body,'" said one new runner who suffered a hamstring injury 6 weeks into a training program. "Well, how can I listen to my body if I don't know what it's telling me?"

There's no easy answer to that, except that experience is by far the best teacher. Longtime runners spend their careers learning to listen to their bodies, with every year making them wiser and more closely attuned to their legs, hearts, and lungs.

It's one of the gifts of running, in fact—this heightened sense of being in tune. Experienced runners understand when they are truly weary versus simply unmotivated. They know what their bodies need and when.

Beyond the hard-earned experience that years of running impart, newcomers can heed the following guidelines to decipher what their bodies are saying.

- **Expect general discomfort at first.** This is the dull, allover soreness of muscles getting used to new work, and chances are you'll feel it not only in your legs but in places you might not expect: arms, neck, shoulders. It takes a whole body to run, and you're using muscles all over that you don't even realize.

    You can take a pain reliever at night or after your run to alleviate this minor discomfort, but don't take such medicines before your next run. This can mask pain, which is the best indicator of how your body is doing.

- **Sharp, specific pain is a sign that something is wrong.** A sudden, localized pain means trouble. That's true whether the pain comes on during or after your run. Sharp pain could be a sign of an acute injury—a muscle pull or bone bruise—or the beginning of an overuse syndrome, such as plantar fasciitis or "runner's knee." Whatever the cause, you should evaluate it.

    What should you do? A good first step for a fairly new runner is to simply take a day or two off. If it's minor, that's all it might need to clear up and go away. If the pain returns after taking a few days off, then it's time to get some professional advice. It's important to try to figure out the underlying cause of the problem; otherwise, it will just return whenever you resume running.

    If the pain is fairly minor, consider a visit to your local running store to ask the experts there to examine your gait and shoes. It might be that your shoes are throwing your feet down in an uncomfortable position. A new pair of shoes or over-the-counter inserts might help.

For more serious pain, a trip to the doctor is in order. A sports medicine physician is the best place to start. These doctors are specifically trained to evaluate sports injuries and serve as gatekeepers to the more specialized world of sports physicians, such as podiatrists and orthopedists. This doctor will let you know if you need to see somebody else or if your problem can be solved with physical therapy or orthotics for your shoes. (For more information on choosing a medical professional for runners, see chapter 8.)

• **Pain that goes away while you're running is not okay.** This type of pain is notorious for fooling runners. An aching hamstring or Achilles tendon feels better after an easy mile of jogging and disappears altogether during the rest of the run. After the run, however, the pain slowly returns, aching even more the next morning, until that day's run magically cures it once again.

The only problem is that you're not curing anything by running. Even though it feels like the running is helping, in fact it's making it worse. What's happening is that some soft-tissue injuries feel better due to the increased motion and bloodflow that occur during running—they are not as tight and, therefore, not giving off pain signals. But once you stop running, the increased trauma takes its toll, resulting in a cycle of deterioration.

These types of injuries—typically muscle strains and tendon inflammations—require a reduction or temporary cessation of running to heal. Running through the injury—even if you swear it feels better during a run—will only exacerbate the problem.

• **Expect discomfort on the comeback trail.** When you resume running after recovering from injury, it's normal once again to have soreness and minor discomfort. You might have scar tissue that is tight and feels different than before, and you probably have lost some overall fitness.

The key is that your discomfort stays just that—not an outright, acute pain—and that it diminishes with each day. If the pain instead becomes more intense, you need to reevaluate your progress. Cut your running in half and build back up more slowly. If you still can't run pain-free, pay another visit to the doctor. You might need more time off to heal or yet a different pair of shoes or orthotics.

RACING REASONABLY

Races are great for beginning runners. They provide a goal for which to train and boost motivation in the process. They're also a great place to meet other runners and enjoy the excitement of the sport. These days, races cater strongly to the "back of the pack" runner, often offering prizes for entertainment and encouragement.

But beginners should approach racing with a certain degree of caution. That's because it's easy to get caught up in the excitement of the event and ignore all the rules of training. That goes for the race itself—and for the training leading up to the event.

When you're training for a race, don't let 1 day of excitement outweigh your wise and cautious long-term training goals. Follow the rules in this chapter and don't train through pain just because your race is a tempting few weeks away. If you do, you risk making an injury worse, perhaps sidelining you for much longer than is necessary.

If your injury requires you to take a few days off to heal, chances are you can still run your race as planned. Just use good judgment to decide. If you've taken a week or more off, you should be okay if the race itself is still several weeks away—you can resume training slowly, and you just won't be in peak condition for the race as you

• **Little things matter.** You might think it's just a tiny blister or a toe bumping up against the front of your shoe, but there's no such thing as an insignificant trauma in running. Repeated running with the same aggravation will only intensify the problem. This in turn can lead to compensation that changes your running form and that can bring on injury somewhere far away from the original source of minor pain.

Always deal with seemingly insignificant traumas and discomforts when you can. If your shoes are tight and causing hot spots, replace them or change the manner in which you are lacing them to alleviate pressure points. If you have a blister, treat it, pad the area around it, and wear different shoes that don't put pressure on the area until it has healed. Heed small pains early on and they won't grow into big problems later.

originally hoped. But ifyou've had to stop running for 2 weeks and now it's a week from race day, it's time to cancel this plan and cheer from the sidelines. You don't want to risk reinjury or a new problem with a sudden hard running effort after such a long layoff. You can always choose a new race to shoot for. It's never worth it to risk injury.

Likewise, if you are in the midst of a race and feel a sudden, severe pain, you might have to call it quits for the day. It's fine to stop, massage the area, and try jogging slowly again to get back in the race—maybe it was just a fleeting pain, a fluke. But if the pain doesn't subside and your running form is compromised, you must give yourself permission to quit the race. Again, there will always be another race. This isn't chickening out—this is called being smart.

Granted, it can be emotionally difficult to change your plans after you've trained for a specific race, to stop in the middle of your adrenaline surge and have to walk off the course. But take the long-term view—always wise in running—and think of all the training and racing to come in your future. It's better to miss 1 day of racing than to miss the next 3 months for a few moments of glory.

• **Avoid running during the heat of the day.** This is especially true when it's very humid. Unconditioned runners are more susceptible to heat illness than conditioned runners. That's because it takes more effort for you to run if you're out of shape (especially if you're overweight), no matter what your speed. High temperature and humidity can eventually take a toll if your body is working so hard that it can no longer cool itself effectively; heat cramps are an early sign of trouble, followed by heat exhaustion.

So if it's hot out when you're first starting your running program, run in the cooler part of the morning or evening. Also be sure that you are well-hydrated. Drink water, juice, or herbal tea throughout the day and drink a glass of sports drink about half an hour before your run and when you finish. (For more on running in the heat, see chapter 7.)

THE MARATHON FOR NEWCOMERS

The marathon is an ancient event, hallowed and mythical. But the classic 26.2-mile footrace has been reborn. Once the sole purview of hardened veterans, marathons now swell with ranks of newcomers.

MORE RUNNING, LESS YOU

Running to lose weight? You've come to the right sport.

Running provides a full-body workout, burning calories at a higher rate than most other exercise. Running stokes the metabolism and dulls the appetite. It builds muscle and burns fat. It requires a minimum amount of time and equipment, making it much easier to stick with than other less convenient exercise programs. Many people first discover running in their attempt to lose weight and then stick with it long after the pounds are shed.

Here are some guidelines for beginners who are running with a goal of slimming down.

Don't "diet" or drastically cut calories. You want to rev up your metabolism, not stall it. Adding a running program is a big change for previously sedentary people, one that requires a source of energy in the form of calories.

The problem with adding workouts and subtracting a lot of calories from your diet at the same time is that you might wind up with an energy deficit. Suddenly, you find yourself exhausted, crabby, and unmotivated. If you're chronically tired, you can bet that the first thing you'll cut from your schedule is your run. And then you're back to square one.

So don't sabotage your efforts by denying your body the energy (which is to say, calories) it needs to exercise properly. Studies have shown that it's more effective to lose weight by burning calories due to increased exercise than simply to cut calories and not exercise. Eat what you need to in order to keep running.

Evaluate your eating habits and gradually make healthy changes. This is different than dieting, which is by nature restrictive and

Perhaps it's no surprise that this distance has taken on such vast popularity. Completing a marathon imparts an unparalleled sense of accomplishment and, with that, converts many folks into committed, long-term runners.

Marathons now also raise tremendous amounts of money for charity.

exclusive. Research has shown again and again that the most effective way to lose weight is to simply eat healthfully and in moderation for a lifetime—not to diet excessively and then binge, Ping-Ponging back and forth between different eating habits.

Strive to get plenty of complex carbohydrates (from whole grains and fresh fruits and vegetables), lean protein (from fish, tofu, legumes, dairy, beef, and chicken), and healthy fats (from nuts, seeds, and olive oil).

So when you start your running program, be kind to your body. Give it the energy it needs to get you through the run. Then let the exercise take the weight off, instead of starving your body.

The bottom line is that the key to weight loss is to expend more calories than you are taking in. All the other minutiae—what time of day you eat, exactly what you eat, and in what order—are relatively insignificant.

Choose your shoes carefully. Make sure you are getting plenty of cushioning and support from your shoes. If you are carrying extra weight, every step results in greater stress on your joints and connective tissues. You might benefit from the beefier shoes on the market that are constructed specifically for heavier runners.

Run on soft surfaces whenever possible. The amount of shock and stress that travels through your body with each footstep is reduced when you run on soft surfaces. Concrete and pavement are more jarring than dirt and wood chips, and they can create a greater risk of injury. When it's possible, take the time to go to a park or path where you can run with less pounding on your joints.

Programs benefiting various foundations funnel thousands of new runners and their pledge dollars toward the marathon each year. These training programs have become one of the primary drivers behind the marathon's evolution from an obscure, hard-core challenge to a mainstream event.

It's a wonderful phenomenon but not without its dangers. The training required to complete a marathon—not to mention the race itself—puts a tremendous amount of stress on the body. Even seasoned runners are at risk for injury. For newcomers, whose bodies are not as conditioned, the marathon must be taken on with great intelligence and patience.

"Don't run a marathon if you're not trained to do so" is the simple, blunt advice from Lewis Maharam, M.D., chairman of the International Marathon Medical Directors Association (IMMDA) Board of Governors and medical director for many of the nation's largest marathons. "Anything can happen, from cardiac to musculoskeletal problems."

While Dr. Maharam doesn't say beginning runners *shouldn't* take on the marathon, he does say that proper preparation is essential.

Here are a few tips for novice runners who've decided to tackle the marathon.

• **Be consistent with your training.** The most important element of marathon training is getting the miles in on your legs. That's the only way for your body to toughen and adapt to the stresses you'll place on it in the marathon race.

• **Don't worry about speed.** Newcomers should run a marathon for completion, not to see how fast they can go. In training, it's more important to run the required number of miles or hours than to do them at a certain speed.

• **Be honest about your training.** Planning on training and actually doing it are two different things. If race day rolls around and you haven't been able to do most of your long runs or if you had to take a month of training off because of a busy work schedule, that means you haven't trained. The wisest course of action is to skip the race. You can't make up lost time running, and you can't "fake it" on race day. It's one thing to go into a 5-K when you're undertrained—the worst that could happen is that you'll slow down—but it's another thing entirely to find yourself in the middle of a marathon and realize you're not prepared. You risk serious injury and exhaustion if you try to push yourself to the finish.

· **Be particularly aware of your fluid intake.** Marathon newbies have been identified as a high-risk category for hyponatremia (low blood sodium), which results when runners take in too much fluid. "This is the most serious issue for the charity marathon runners," Dr. Maharam says. "It's their first marathon, they hear the old wives' tale that they need to drink and drink and drink. It's not true."

The problem is that most new runners will not be going fast enough to spill tremendous amounts of sweat. By drinking too much replacement fluid, they risk becoming hyponatremic, a dangerous condition that can lead to organ failure and, in extreme cases, death. The problem is particularly confounding because new runners have long been admonished to drink as much as possible. In addition, the symptoms of hyponatremia mimic those of dehydration, making it hard to distinguish the two without a blood test.

Dr. Maharam says there's a simple solution, and it's the one now advocated by the IMMDA. Instead of drinking as much as possible, runners are advised to drink according to their thirst. So don't guzzle endlessly—if you're thirsty, drink; if you're not, don't force it. That's the best hydration formula for new marathoners and the best advice for a successful first marathon. (For more on dehydration and hyponatremia, see chapter 7.)

12

YOUNG RUNNERS

LOOKING TOWARD THE FUTURE

Before discussing any risks children might undertake by running, a strong statement of perspective is in order: The dangers of children not participating in sports—athletics in general or running specifically—far outweigh the dangers of participating.

Children in the United States are overweight and underexercised. Obesity has become an epidemic; in fact, it's the number one health concern facing our children today, according to numerous health organizations. In turn, as overweight children grow up to be overweight adults, obesity-related health problems such as high cholesterol, heart disease, and diabetes are reaching record proportions.

The problem stems from myriad causes, first and foremost atrocious nutrition practices and the insidious popularity of sedentary pursuits such as video and computer games. The solution must target the numerous causes. In other words, we need to overhaul our societal attitudes about what we eat and how we fill up our spare time. Meanwhile, as part of the solution, encouraging children to participate in sports and exercise can go a long way toward addressing the weight problems they face.

Sports get kids outside and moving around. The physical activity burns calories, but it does more than that. Sports foster discipline and teamwork. They build self-esteem and positive body image. Studies have shown that even the dangers of drugs and early sexual encounters are less of an issue for youngsters who take part in sports. Finally, getting into the habit of exercising early in life translates into good health habits later on.

The best way to get your child interested in sports is to set a positive example yourself. Toddlers are masters of imitation—they'll often mimic Mommy or Daddy stretching, running, even icing their legs. If children grow up knowing that athletics is something their parents do every day, then chances are they'll believe it's something they should be doing, too. And that's one of the best things you can do for your child's health.

THE BUDDING RUNNER

If your child has shown an interest in running, your mission now is to keep him or her enthusiastic and healthy. The best way to accomplish that is not to go overboard by encouraging intense training or competition. Make your child's running goals fun-based, rather than performance-based. Achieving maximal gains in the sport should not be a priority. In fact, most experts agree that youngsters should not engage in serious training until high school. And even then, long-term health and fitness should be the primary driver, not high school stardom.

Experts suggest that the best athletic program for youngsters through the middle school years is one that allows them to experiment in many areas. Ideally, children should participate in several sports throughout the year, perhaps one each season.

The renaissance approach is recommended for all children, but for young runners in particular. Running does not require prodigies of tender age, unlike gymnastics or figure skating, which demand a tremendous degree of flexibility, skill, and fearlessness, abilities that tend to peak during or shortly after childhood. Running skills typically develop over time—years, even decades, of conditioning the body. In fact, runners who have competed at the world-class level have picked up the sport at all ages, including well into adulthood.

Here are five specific reasons children should avoid specializing in one sport to the exclusion of others.

Burnout. Children who engage in a sport earnestly can rapidly use up their well of excitement. Even if they show talent and enthusiasm early on, their motivation can quickly flag. They run the risk of growing bored or even starting to dislike their sport before reaching their potential. Research has shown that children who specialize in a sport before puberty tend to have shorter sports "careers" than those who wait until after puberty to focus.

Injury. The American Podiatric Medical Association, in its statement on children and sports, says that children who specialize in a single sport at a young age are more likely to develop foot and ankle injuries. In running, in particular, the injury rate for youngsters is directly related to the number of hours they devote to the sport. Injury is not only a health issue for children but also a psychological risk, since it can quickly dampen their enthusiasm.

Variety staves off injury by reducing trauma and stress to any one particular area. Throughout middle school, children shouldn't engage in anything that could be construed as "training." Rather, children should treat running as play. In high school, training should be moderate and approached with caution. For more on appropriate running levels for different ages, see the sidebar on pages 164 and 165.

Broad athletic skill development. Youth is the best time to develop and master a variety of physical skills—throwing a curveball, for example, swimming the butterfly stroke, or dribbling a soccer ball. Just as there is a window of opportunity for learning language when a child is young, sports that involve specific coordination requirements are best served by an introduction at a young age when the body is most accommodating to learning new movements. Remember, there's no hurry for running. Running is something children and adults can always discover or return to, since little to no technique is involved. And since serious training is best reserved for later years, your child will enjoy greater health benefits by participating in other sports.

Peaking too soon. Runners who train seriously will naturally improve. Then, after several years, the gains stop coming so easily. If your child shows potential and hopes to be a star in college or even go on with hopes of a professional career, patience will be her greatest attribute. The number of "years on your legs" clearly takes a toll for runners later in life. And the running world is filled with anonymous former "bright, young hopefuls" who were never heard from again after high school. This is not to say that youngsters can't run and even race, but the level of intensity should be moderate.

(continued on page 166)

PLAYING VERSUS TRAINING

How much can children safely run at each age? There's no magic formula or official guideline, says Jordan Metzl, M.D., medical director of the Sports Medicine Institute for Young Athletes at the Hospital for Special Surgery in New York City. He does use the following rules of thumb for the maximum amount a child should run at any given time (but not every day).

- Under age 10: 3.2 miles (or about 30 minutes)
- Under age 12: 6.4 miles (or about 60 minutes)
- Under age 14: 10 miles (or about 90 minutes)

Children under the age of 12 are advised to run no more than three or four times a week; children under the age of 14 should run no more than four or five times a week. Beyond that, here are some guidelines for the healthy, active development of your future runner at various stages.

Toddler/preschool. Children this age will often want to imitate Mom and Dad and their own friends, so it's an important time to set a good example.

Kids' races are a terrific way to make children feel a part of things and to introduce them to the sport. But, again, keep the emphasis on fun. Don't ever force them to participate. Toddlers are notorious for changing their minds; they might be jumping with excitement all morning and then balk on the starting line. If they decide after the gun goes off that they don't want to run, don't force the issue.

Also be sure to choose races that are an appropriate distance for your child. Don't trust race organizers to know what that distance is. Just because they're offering a mile open to all ages doesn't mean your little one can or should go that far. Generally speaking, children ages 2 and 3 are best off with little "dashes" of 100 yards. Most 4- and 5-year-olds can comfortably handle a quarter-mile; some can do half a mile. Use your judgment and don't exceed your child's natural inclination.

Grade school and middle school. Grade school is the time for children to explore with sports. If they love running, that's great, but don't push them to "train" by running a certain number of minutes or miles per day. Instead, they can have informal races with friends and siblings, running around the block or the park. Encourage other fun sports that require running, such as soccer.

By the age of 11 or 12, your child might want to run in a more organized effort. Limit most runs to 2 or 3 miles (typically 20 to 30 minutes) at a time, no more than four times a week. Once a week, kids could go a little longer, up to 5 or 6 miles (up to 60 minutes) if they desire. Look for a soft surface for them to run on—grass or cinders—whenever possible.

When it comes to racing, be extra careful not to exceed your child's abilities. Races of a mile or so are best for early grade school. A 5-K or 10-K will be possible for some children by middle school, but explain to them that they might have to walk part of the way—and then plan to jog and walk with them in the race so that they're not alone. Chances are they'll be fine during the race, but your presence will be of great comfort should they find themselves overextended and unsure how to proceed. (If they do exhaust themselves early in the race, walk to the finish or, depending on the course, find the nearest shortcut back to your car, home, or starting area.)

High school. This is when most young runners begin to train in earnest. Not surprisingly, it's also when many of them become frustrated by a string of injuries.

Just like any other runners, youngsters must follow the laws of training outlined earlier in this book: increasing mileage and intensity very gradually and methodically. Many high school injuries can be traced to a sudden surge of running after a period of inactivity. Youngsters can reduce the chance of injury by preparing for running seasons in advance, starting with some very slow, easy mileage weeks before joining the team for training.

How much should a high school child run? Training for freshman and sophomore high school runners should be about 15 to 25 miles a week. Upperclassmen can handle slightly more, up to about 35 miles a week. But these are only guidelines. If a child is unenthusiastic or injury-prone, chances are he's running too much.

TOO YOUNG FOR THE DISTANCE?

In the fall of 2001, the International Marathon Medical Directors Association (IMMDA) approved this advisory statement: "Marathon running should be reserved only for those individuals who have reached their 18th birthday." Most marathons have adopted the recommendations of the IMMDA and accordingly raised the entry age to 18. Here are some of the many reasons why the marathon and the young runner are not a good mix.

• Young runners competing at their typical high school distance of no more than 3 miles already suffer from a high rate of injury. A young person training to run more than eight times that distance is just begging for trouble.

• Children have a harder time dissipating heat and a lower capacity to sweat, increasing the danger of developing heat illness during long endurance events such as the marathon.

• Children might suffer psychological and emotional problems, such as frustration and feeling like a failure, if they take on an event that exceeds their natural abilities.

If your young runner has been bitten by the marathon bug, help her to realize that this is one goal best saved for later.

Changing body types. Before puberty, it's impossible to tell how a child's body will develop. A youngster who says, "I'm going to be a distance runner" ultimately might be disappointed as large muscle mass develops that makes him more adept for shot putting, football, or triathlons. By maintaining an interest in a variety of sports, children are less likely to become disappointed in their sports—and their bodies. They are also more likely to discover the sport that they enjoy most or at which they are most successful.

SPECIAL INJURY CONCERNS

Running ranks high on the list of sports that induce injuries. One notorious Seattle-area study conducted over many years delivered the sobering news that girls' cross-country produced the highest injury rate of any high school sport—higher even than traditional contact sports such as football and wrestling. Boys' cross-country came in fifth, behind these three sports and girls' soccer.

In almost any sport in which girls and boys both participate, girls suffer more injuries. So it should come as no surprise that girl runners suffer injury at a rate that is estimated to be anywhere from two times to eight times that of boys. The reason may be due to several factors, including poorer presports conditioning, wider hips that lead to greater knee troubles, and weaker bone density, sometimes caused by menstrual irregularities.

Why does running take such a toll on young runners? "The thing to understand is that running is a contact sport—between you and the ground," says Stephen Rice, Ph.D., the pediatric sports specialist who conducted the groundbreaking study.

The impact forces of running are a compounded problem for children, whose bones are not yet fully developed. Soft cartilage growth plates, which don't close until the age of 15 or so, are more susceptible to the tremendous forces of running. Also, bone growth tends to occur in spurts unrelated to the elongation of connective tissue, which often lags behind, resulting in imbalances and inflexibility. The soft, developing bones become particularly vulnerable to these imbalances, making them an easy target for injury.

At the base of it, though, many children's injuries are preventable, just as injuries in adults are preventable. That's because the reason for injury at any age is basically the same: too much stress on a body that is not conditioned for it—in other words, overuse. Because children have the added vulnerability of growing bones and connective tissue, they have to be that much more careful not to overdo it.

To avoid injury, then, parents and children must exercise caution and pay close attention to early warning signs of trauma, such as soreness and muscle tightness. "The threshold for getting a child investigated should be slightly less than for an adult," says Jordan Metzl, M.D., medical director of the Sports Medicine Institute for Young Athletes at the Hospital for Special Surgery in New York City. In other words, while an adult might wait a week and self-treat to see how an ache progresses, 2 to 3 days is the limit before getting medical attention for a child.

Early intervention is especially important at a young age because running injuries tend to become chronic, and one injury is a strong predictor of future injury. Proper treatment can prevent injuries way down the line, Dr. Metzl says. An Achilles tendon that becomes tender during childhood can bother a person well into adulthood.

COMMON YOUTH INJURIES

Most overuse injuries occur when kids reach high school, the time they start training in earnest for track or cross-country. Three of the most common injuries suffered by young runners are:

Shin splints. This is actually a general, nonmedical term that refers to pain in the shin area. According to Dr. Metzl, the problem can be either muscular or bone-related. In either case, microtrauma occurs, causing pain in the shin area. In some cases, it's because of over-pronation, which places excess stress along the tibia. The bone can become inflamed, and the condition can eventually cause a stress fracture. Muscular pain on the outside of the shin might instead be due to *compartment syndrome,* in which the muscle does not have adequate room to expand.

No matter what the source, the key is to address shin pain in young runners immediately. "In almost every case, this is not only treatable but also fully preventable," Dr. Metzl says. He recommends a visit to a sports medicine physician, who can analyze the runner's biomechanics, training, and diet and determine a proper course of action.

Some reduction of training might be necessary until the pain disappears. And the doctor might determine that a good pair of motion-control running shoes is required or an over-the-counter arch insert to control excessive pronation.

Osgood-Schlatter syndrome. Felt as pain just under the kneecap, Osgood-Schlatter syndrome is caused by a disparity in the growth rate of bone and tendon (see above). The tugging that occurs at the bone-tendon attachment during periods of bone growth can cause trauma to the soft cartilage growth plates.

A temporary reduction of training might be necessary until the tendon-bone imbalance works itself out. This would be a good time for cross-training (see chapter 6); limiting the amount of running will alleviate the trauma in the knee area. Meanwhile, ice can reduce some of the associated pain.

Stress fractures. Children are more prone than adults to stress fractures, because they face a double whammy with every step they take. First, their still-developing bones are soft and vulnerable to impact forces. Second, because children are smaller and have a shorter stride, they must take more steps to cover the same distance—thus multiplying the repetition of stress and impact.

Stress fractures require time off from running until they are healed. An injury of this nature should also be considered a strong invitation to review and improve the young athlete's diet. A susceptibility to stress fractures might be an indication of poor nutrition. Children today consume fewer dairy products and more soda and caffeine than previous generations, both of which hamper the development of bone mass. Young athletes should be sure to consume sources of calcium, including dairy products, calcium-fortified juices, leafy green vegetables, and fish.

What You Can Do

All these injuries—and most others that strike young runners—are primarily due to overuse. The key to avoiding them is to train within reasonable limits and take some preventive measures.

Always increase training gradually. Children must be especially careful to follow the laws of proper training, first gradually building a base and only then adding faster, more intense running. Like adults, they can use the 10 percent guideline, increasing training distance or intensity by only 10 percent in any given week.

Youngsters are especially prone to injury when they begin training at the start of cross-country or track season, particularly if they have not been running much over the summer or winter break. Be sure they communicate their current level of conditioning to the coach and then work together to develop an appropriate program. Track and cross-country camps in particular are notorious for placing heavy training loads on unconditioned athletes; youngsters should prepare with some running and other activity in the weeks or months ahead of time.

Following is a sample training schedule for a high school freshman or sophomore preparing for fall cross-country season. Upperclassmen who run year-round and are more likely to be conditioned can start this schedule at a base of 30 minutes, 4 days a week. This training should be conducted in the 6 weeks *leading up to* the start of formal practice.

	WEEK 1	WEEK 2	WEEK 3	WEEK 4	WEEK 5	WEEK 6
MONDAY	20 min.	20 min.	20 min.	20 min.	20 min.	20 min.
TUESDAY	20 min.	25 min.	25 min.	30 min.	30 min., plus 3 or 4 strides slightly up-tempo for 50–100 yards	30 min., plus 5 or 6 strides slightly up-tempo for 50–100 yards
WEDNESDAY	rest	rest	rest	rest	rest	rest
THURSDAY	20 min.	20 min.	20 min.	20 min.	20 min.	20 min.
FRIDAY	rest or swim/bike	rest or swim/bike	rest or swim/bike	rest or swim/bike	rest or swim/bike	rest or swim/bike
SATURDAY	20 min.	25 min.	30 min.	35 min.	40 min.	40 min., with last 5 min. slightly up-tempo
SUNDAY	rest	rest	rest	rest	rest	rest

Pay attention to early warning signs. Aches and pains should be heeded and treated, not ignored or "run through." Traditional PRICE (protection, rest, ice, compression, and elevation) treatment can help reduce inflammation and pain early in the course of many injuries. (See chapter 8 for more details.) Training levels should be reduced before the injury becomes severe. And a sports medicine specialist should be consulted if pain persists. If your child tends to be uncommunicative, you might not be aware of the warning signs, even an outright injury, unless you ask. In addition to obvious signals like limping or swelling, signs that something is amiss include a loss of enthusiasm for training and making excuses for missing a workout.

Make sure your child eats a wholesome diet with adequate calcium. Because of bone vulnerability, calcium intake is particularly important. Studies show some grim trends. It's estimated that only one in five children consumes the recommended daily amount of calcium, which is 1,300 milligrams for children ages 9 to 18. (Children ages 4 to 8 should consume roughly 800 milligrams.) Meanwhile, bone fractures in children have increased markedly in the past few decades.

"The amount of milk that kids drink has decreased over the past 15 years, and the amount of soda they consume has increased," Dr. Metzl says. The two simultaneous trends spell trouble for kids who run. "I never used to see kids with stress fractures, and now I do," he says. Not only that, but children with already low bone density are setting themselves up for osteoporosis later in life. That's because the body builds bone only during youth; after age 30, we are incapable of boosting bone density.

Low-fat milk remains the best source of calcium. It's fortified with vitamin D, which is necessary for the absorption of calcium, and it also contains fat and protein. Fortified juices, while they do provide calcium, generally lack these other essentials—although some juices now contain D. Additional sources include other dairy products such as cheese and yogurt. Tofu, dark leafy vegetables, and canned salmon and sardines also contain calcium. Children who are picky eaters can take a supplement as insurance that they'll get enough calcium.

Cross-train, particularly with strengthening exercises. Since children are often interested in many activities anyway, cross-training is a natural way to prevent injuries. Allow or encourage your kids to participate in numerous sports. The variety your child engages in when younger needn't stop in high school just because she's on the track team.

Cross-training can accomplish several things.

• It can provide overall conditioning, since young runners must limit the amount of actual running they do.

• It builds muscle strength, which is crucial for supporting the skeleton and shielding joints from the impact forces of running.

• Weight-bearing activities, weight lifting in particular, also develop bone strength. (True, running is a weight-bearing activity. But since there is a limit to how much a child should run, the answer to proper conditioning for children is cross-training.) Dr. Metzl recommends that children engage in regular (but not overly strenuous) strength training starting as early as age 8 or 9. Simple exercises with light dumbbells or weight machines are the safest. For an individualized workout, ask whether local schools, recreation centers, YMCAs, or athletic clubs know of trainers who specialize in youth fitness. Trainers can be certified by several different organizations, the most reputable being the American College of Sports Medicine (ACSM) and the American Council on Exercise. Look for a trainer with a degree in exercise science or a health-related field, such as kinesiology. The

HYDRATION FOR YOUNG RUNNERS

Young runners are more likely to become dehydrated than adults. The reasons are numerous.

• Children have a lesser ability to generate sweat.

• They have a higher ratio of body mass to surface area, meaning they can't dissipate heat as efficiently.

• They are not as conscientious as adults about drinking during or before activity.

These factors can combine to exacerbate the dangers of dehydration for young runners. Parents need to be aware and encourage hydration.

Youngsters should drink to stay hydrated throughout the day, not just during or after runs or races. Active youngsters should drink at least 8 to 10 ounces of water or other liquid at breakfast, lunch, and dinner, as well as before and after any workouts.

Young runners should drink shortly before races or workouts. They should aim to drink 5 to 10 ounces of water or sports drink every 20 minutes during workouts (the lesser amount for children under 100 pounds and the higher amount for children over 100 pounds). And they should always drink copiously after runs and races.

Since children drink less when they are consuming plain water, let them drink a sports drink or diluted juice during or after activity. (Because these tend to contain large amounts of sugar, parents might not want to make these available any time of day. Reserving them for athletic use is a good compromise.)

ACSM Web site can help you find a trainer in your area with its ProFinder feature; go to www.acsm.org. Ask for references and check certifications.

Stretch regularly after running. Stretching is particularly important for adolescents. While younger children are extremely flexible, this tends to decrease in adolescence, when rapid skeletal growth leaves muscles and connective tissue shorter in relation to bone and therefore tight and inflexible. Junior high and high school runners should stretch regularly after runs as part of their conditioning. The stretches in chapter 4 are appropriate for young runners. Youngsters should be cautioned not to turn stretching into a competitive exercise—the goal is not to see who can stretch the farthest but to stretch only to the point of mild resistance.

Invest in running shoes for your child. It's not a lot of equipment, after all, and will cost you far less than outfitting a child for, say, ice hockey. Buy running-specific shoes, since general tennis shoes do not offer adequate protection. And plan to buy new ones every year or even twice a year—kids' feet grow fast! Many running specialty stores and large sporting goods stores now carry running shoes for children.

13

WOMEN RUNNERS

SPECIAL HEALTH ISSUES

Back in the dark ages of running (anytime before about 1980), women were considered simply not up to the physical requirements of the sport. Their bodies and psyches were too fragile, it was believed. Running harms the reproductive system, it was thought. Or injures just about any part of a woman's body. Or causes the development of masculine attributes. A whole host of old wives' tales emerge about the ill effects of running, which had the perhaps intentional effect of discouraging women from the sport.

Today, we know that there is no truth to any of this. Women now compete at distances and intensities that match those of men. The best women runners can easily trounce upward of 99 percent of the men on the planet. And even among recreational runners, women's bodies—and brains—have proven more than adequate for the rigors of the sport.

That's not to say that there are no differences between male and female athletes. Women's reproductive systems create unique health concerns during pregnancy and postpartum. And during their lives, women's hormones fluctuate to a greater degree than those of men, creating additional health issues. Female body composition in general differs in many ways from that of men. Women have less bone and muscle mass, smaller hearts, more body fat, and greater elasticity in their connective tissue. Their hips and pelvises are wider, and they tend to pronate to a greater degree than men.

All of these factors mean that many women have significant risk factors for injury. But women runners are in no way *guaranteed* to get hurt. Women can prevent injury the same way any other runner can: by training properly and paying close attention to body mechanics and how they relate to proper footwear and care.

KNEE PROBLEMS

Much has been made of the fact that women's knees are more vulnerable to injury than those of men. Research that exposed the prevalence of anterior cruciate ligament (ACL) tears among girls and women made headlines, but the exact implications of the findings are still not clear. That's because the reasons for the high rate of injury to this tissue in the knee joint are not fully understood. Is it simply a matter of women's body shape, their wider pelvises, and the resulting inward knee rotation? Is it that women tend to be less conditioned in general, and a lack of strength in the tissues supporting the knee makes it vulnerable? Or is it that women's connective tissue is more lax and flexible, an inherent weakness that would be difficult to correct? In fact, the high rate of ACL tears in women could be due to some combination of all these factors and more.

These particular injuries occur mostly in women who play such sports as soccer and basketball, which require players to stop suddenly or land abruptly after jumping. Runners, on the other hand, move along at a steady pace, with no such ballistic movements. So, it's typically not running itself that causes the problem. However, it turns out that the same anatomical and conditioning factors that predispose women to outright ACL tears might also make them highly vulnerable to another type of knee injury, patellofemoral pain syndrome, or runner's knee.

Here's what we can safely say about women runners and their knees.

• Women runners do indeed frequently suffer knee pain and knee injury.

• Pain and injury can be due to several different factors, including misalignment, strength imbalances, connective tissue factors, previous trauma, improper footwear, and just plain overtraining.

What You Can Do

Assess your biomechanics. If you suffer from knee aggravation, your course of treatment should be no different than that of a male runner. Namely, you should have your biomechanics analyzed by a sports physician, professional trainer, or physical therapist. In virtually all cases of knee injury, some underlying mechanical issue is at work. Many of these problems can be corrected with proper footwear or shoe inserts.

Get stronger. Strengthening exercises are particularly helpful for knee injuries and can alleviate many problems. A physical therapist or trainer should analyze muscle strength in your leg, trunk, hips, and pelvic area and then prescribe specific exercises. It's better to work with a trained professional to develop an individual strength-training program than to embark on a generic strength program yourself. That's because, for knee injuries, you need to focus on correcting imbalances among muscle groups, rather than overall strength.

Train smart. Finally, always increase training gradually, as discussed throughout this book. Knee injuries, like all overuse injuries, tend to surface when your training threshold has been surpassed too quickly.

BONE HEALTH

Bone health is a far more insidious health concern for women than for men. That's because the female hormone estrogen, which protects bone strength by regulating calcium absorption, fluctuates to a greater degree in women's bodies than the comparable male hormone, testosterone, does in men. After menopause, when estrogen production slows, bone loss can accelerate dramatically.

Weight-bearing exercise—including running—has been conclusively shown to help maintain bone density. That's because, as with muscle, exercise that stresses the bones prompts a conditioning response that strengthens them. In bone, this occurs on a cellular level, as osteoblasts (immature bone cells) are stimulated in response to stress; these in turn secrete proteins that eventually crystallize into bone. Indeed, a sedentary lifestyle is considered one of the risk factors for osteoporosis, the medical term for the weakening of the bones that makes them susceptible to fracture.

But there's a downside to running in terms of bone health. Some female runners, particularly younger competitive ones, develop disordered eating patterns in conjunction with their athletic endeavors. Insufficient nutrition and caloric intake can result in a chain of connected health issues: extremely low body fat, hormonal imbalances, and menstrual dysfunction. All these directly compromise bone health—remember that bone loss is linked to hormone production—often leading to osteoporosis in even very young runners. If they are very thin, even runners who don't have actual eating disorders might be compromising their bone health due to decreased estrogen levels (the hormone's production is linked to body fat).

Compromised bone health is a serious issue and not one reserved for the elderly. Young, athletic women with brittle bones are susceptible to stress fractures. Older women are at risk of outright bone fractures, which have been linked to a host of other complications that can depress the quality and even length of life.

What You Can Do

Start early and keep at it. Maintaining good bone health is a lifetime proposition. Here's why. Your body accrues most of its bone mass in your teens and twenties. In fact, it's estimated that 90 percent of total bone mineral content is deposited during adolescence, a small window of opportunity that's soon closed. By the age of 30, your body has achieved maximum bone density, and it declines slowly from there.

The speed of that decline depends on a number of risk factors. Some are in your control, for example, calcium intake, exercise, and avoiding excessive caffeine, alcohol, and soda. (Carbonated beverages contain phosphorus, which gets in the way of calcium absorption.) Factors that are beyond your control include heredity, your menstrual patterns, and the onset of menopause. And you might be surprised to hear that some medications and medical conditions can adversely affect bone density, including thyroid disease, hysterectomy, antacids that contain aluminum (it also interferes with calcium absorption), and prednisone.

What does it mean to you? That at every stage of life you can be contributing either to your bones' health or to their demise. In your teens and twenties, you should be laying the foundation for solid bones that must last the rest of your life. From age 30 on, you're working to maintain as much of that density as possible.

Pay attention to your diet. It's crucial at any age to consume a healthy diet that contains adequate calcium. Magnesium and vitamins C and D also help, since they aid in absorption of calcium. Dairy products, soy products, fish, fresh fruits and vegetables, beans, whole grains, and calcium-fortified juices should be part of the daily diet. Minimize your intake of soda, caffeine, alcohol, and high-fat processed foods, since these can leach minerals from bone.

Exercise. Weight-bearing activities, such as running and weight lifting, are vital throughout your life—from your youth through and beyond menopause. The strengthening effect of exercise is most pronounced during youth, but continued activity remains an important factor in maintaining bone strength as you age.

Get your bones tested. If you have risk factors for osteoporosis, undergo testing to determine your bone density. If osteoporosis is diagnosed, a physician and nutritionist can assess your dietary habits and lifestyle. Your doctor may prescribe medication in severe cases of osteoporosis.

Finally, any time you suffer a stress fracture, you should have the overall health of your bones assessed. This will help to determine whether the fracture was an isolated incident due to training overload or if your bone health is indeed compromised to a degree that requires nutritional and lifestyle evaluation.

RUNNING AND THE MENSTRUAL CYCLE

Running itself does not disrupt a woman's menstrual functioning. However, intense running in conjunction with other factors, particularly inadequate nutrition, can lead to a disruption or even cessation of menstruation.

Menstrual dysfunction can take different forms, including a delayed onset of an adolescent's period, a diminished number of cycles (oligomenorrhea), an absence of periods altogether (amenorrhea), and the absence of ovulation even when the rest of the menstrual cycle appears normal (anovulation).

Absent periods are not a good thing. Some female runners are guilty of viewing amenorrhea as a sign of tremendous fitness, believing that it means they're at a lean, fighting weight. While it's true that thin runners perform better than overweight ones, this idea often is taken too far.

When the body does not have enough fat reserves to function properly, it begins operating in survival mode, and it's only a matter of time before running performance and overall health decline. At this point, the body considers fertility a luxury and effectively shuts it down. As discussed in the previous section on bone health, an inadequate diet and compromised hormonal function are direct causes of osteoporosis, which is a serious health issue. Even when proper menstrual functioning is restored, any loss of bone density that occurs will never be completely reversible.

If premature bone thinning isn't enough to convince a competitive runner that menstrual dysfunction is something to be concerned about, she might eventually be forced to look at it this way: The stress fractures that inevitably result will stop her running in its tracks.

The other drawback of menstrual irregularities is that they obviously make getting pregnant difficult or impossible. In the case of menstrual difficulties that are linked to athletics, most of the impact on fertility is believed to be reversible. However, it can take time to restore proper menstrual functioning and fertility.

What You Can Do

See a doctor. While intense exercise often correlates with menstrual irregularities, never assume that such dysfunction is due to athletics. You need to have a physician rule out other intrinsic causes that might have nothing to do with your training; for example, hypothyroidism or ovarian disease.

Consider your energy equation. In the past, running alone was considered the culprit in a runner's menstrual dysfunction. Today, the more accepted reasoning is that running is just one factor in what can be called your "energy equation." On the left side of the equation are adequate nutrition, caloric intake, and rest. On the right side are your stress levels, body composition, and the amount of running you do. If the factors on the right add up to more than the amount of rest you get and your nutritional profile, your body goes into deficit mode.

Running is just part of the equation, which means that you needn't necessarily cut back your training to reestablish normal menstrual functioning. In most cases, boosting the other side of the equation by making dietary adjustments to meet your caloric expenditure can do the trick. In other words, you have to eat enough.

There's more to it, of course. "[Female runners] need to counteract running with rest and good diet and a good psychological outlook on life," says Christine Wells, Ph.D., professor emerita of exercise science and physical education at Arizona State University. You also need to counter what Dr. Wells calls "an addiction atmosphere," in which you are driven not only to run to excess but to curtail eating as well. Because there are so many factors involved in your energy equation, if you're concerned about menstrual irregularities, your best plan of action is to work with a team of trusted professionals, including a general sports medicine physician, a gynecologist, a nutritionist, and a sports therapist.

DIETARY ISSUES

Chances are you've heard of anorexia and bulimia, which are severe and debilitating eating disorders. Highly competitive female athletes—particularly those in high school and college—are prone to such diseases, especially in sports in which thinness is an attribute. (Yes, that includes running.) These illnesses are very serious, even life threatening, but are also fairly rare.

But not every eating disorder is so dramatic or, in fact, particularly rare. A far more common problem exists among female runners, one that cuts across a wider swath of ages and competitive abilities. Disordered eating, as it has come to be called, while not immediately life threatening, is debilitating and deceptive.

Disordered eating can manifest itself in many different ways. Some women count calories obsessively, restricting overall eating to a minimum. Others eliminate specific food groups from their diet, shunning fats, breads, or sweets. Sometimes, women exercise fanatically solely to burn calories in an attempt to offset what they have eaten. The obsessions can change from year to year, fluctuating in degree and severity as an athlete tries to control her weight and body. Some women with disordered eating eventually develop full-fledged eating disorders, while others maintain a low level of disorder.

According to the American College of Sports Medicine, up to 62 percent of female college athletes report a history of some manner of disordered eating. Athletes are at higher risk than the general population, and while disordered eating peaks in young adulthood, some women suffer such problems their entire life.

Disordered eating is one of the three corners on a triangle of inter-related issues that has come to be known as Female Athlete Triad. The three aspects of the triad are disordered eating, menstrual irregularities, and osteoporosis. Often found in conjunction and difficult to separate, they present serious health problems for the female athlete. As mentioned above, an overly restrictive diet is often a direct cause of poor bone health and menstrual irregularities. Other dangers of restricted eating include gastrointestinal difficulties and cardiovascular abnormalities.

What You Can Do

Disordered eating and outright eating disorders should not be ignored. The sooner restrictive dietary habits are identified and addressed, the more easily they are treated, since patterns won't yet have become as ingrained.

Seek professional help. Anorexia and bulimia should not be self-treated alone. They are a serious health issue requiring professional treatment. A physician or nutritionist can refer a patient or family to the proper local resources or to a national organization that specializes in such matters.

Take a multidimensional approach. Treating disordered eating is a matter of degrees. In many cases, the runner will still benefit from professional treatment. Because disordered eating is both a mental and a physical issue, approaching treatment from several angles is often most effective. Consult with:

• A **physician** to monitor bone density and general health

• A **nutritionist,** who can devise a healthy eating plan

• A **therapist** or **psychiatrist** for help with emotional factors, including depression, perfectionist tendencies, family difficulties, or pressure to perform

• The **coach,** who can monitor training schedules (In the case of younger athletes, some coaches and parents will not allow the athlete to train unless she is at a healthy weight.)

• The **parents** or **spouse** for general support

Change your attitude. In general, the focus must be to rethink attitudes toward food. Women runners with disordered eating patterns tend to view food as the enemy, something that must be controlled and defeated. It is helpful instead to view food as an ally in performance, since it provides the fuel that is required for optimal training. Often, underlying emotional issues that might have nothing to do with food or athletics—depression or family dynamics—must be dealt with as well.

RUNNING AND FERTILITY

Running at a recreational level does not adversely affect fertility. In addition, recreational runners are more likely to take better care of themselves in general—with good nutrition and minimal exposure to smoking and alcohol. That means that running is a positive activity overall for women who are attempting to conceive (and not a bad thing for their partners, either).

Difficulties with fertility usually arise in women who are training at a highly competitive level—those who train every day or even twice a day. As discussed in the section on menstrual irregularities above, an overall energy deficit can occur in some highly athletic women, causing the body to dial down its nonessential systems. Resulting menstrual inconsistencies can lead to infertility. The problem isn't just that these women are running hard but that their training isn't balanced with adequate rest and nutrition.

What You Can Do

Eat and sleep. Menstrual irregularities that are related to athletics are typically easy to reverse with adequate nutrition and rest.

Slow down. If you are actively attempting to become pregnant, cutting back training temporarily is a sensible course of action. After all, during pregnancy, competition is no longer the primary goal, and intense, high-mileage training isn't necessary. You can decrease your overall mileage and curtail highly intense speed workouts. If you've been competing at a very lean body mass, it won't hurt to gain a few pounds.

See a doctor. As mentioned previously, menstrual difficulties actually might not be linked to running. Women experiencing fertility challenges should not assume that training is the culprit and should receive proper medical attention to address the issue.

RUNNING DURING PREGNANCY

Running during pregnancy is not only safe but also beneficial for mothers—and possibly even babies. Here are just some of the positive impacts of regular exercise.

- Less excessive weight gain

- Higher energy level and improved mood and attitude

- Less overall discomfort and back pain

- Better physical conditioning for mothers to deal with and recover from labor and delivery

- Shorter labor with fewer complications

- More rapid weight loss after delivery

- A possible decrease in the incidence of preterm births and low-birth-weight babies

If this information comes as a surprise, it might be because women traditionally have been advised to cease strenuous activity during pregnancy. They were told to keep their heart rate below 140 beats per minute during exercise. Running in particular was thought to be especially bad, since it was believed to stress the mother unduly—and jiggle the baby, to boot.

The American College of Obstetrics and Gynecology revised its guidelines for exercise in the mid 1990s. When it did so, it eliminated heart rate and duration targets, instead advising pregnant women to gauge their effort based on how they feel while exercising, or perceived exertion.

Heart rate, long considered to be the reliable indicator of effort during pregnancy, was discarded in part because it turned out to be a poor barometer of effort. For one thing, heart rate changes dramatically during pregnancy, increasing even without exertion. Additionally, too much variety exists among women based on heredity, level of conditioning, and age. Many women found that there was no way they could exercise even minimally without exceeding 140 beats per minute.

Of course, pregnant women do need to take precautions. Training to exhaustion and overheating are still not advised. But it's generally accepted that women with healthy pregnancies can safely engage in moderate exercise. Unlike in the past, when exercise was approached with fearful trepidation, pregnant women now can safely be counseled to listen to and trust their bodies.

One helpful way to think of running during pregnancy is to focus on the shift in priorities. Before pregnancy, your goal might have been maximum fitness for yourself. During pregnancy, it becomes optimal health for you *and* your baby. That means you shouldn't be "training" per se but running moderately in order to remain healthy. This change in attitude can help you make appropriate exercise choices. The idea isn't to run as much or as hard as possible but just to get out and get some exercise.

What You Can Do

• Exercise up to a moderate level based on your perceived exertion.

• Take care not to overheat; wear layers so that you can moderate your temperature and do not exercise in excessive heat or humidity.

• Exercising most days of the week is preferable to sporadic bouts of exercise.

• Consider running on smooth, obstacle-free surfaces, such as cinder tracks, rather than on trails. Increases in joint laxity due to pregnancy hormones might make strains or sprains more likely.

• Drink often to stay well-hydrated.

• Be sure to visit your health practitioner regularly and consult with her about your level of exercise. For example, inadequate weight gain by you or your baby might be a sign that you're exercising too much.

• After the first trimester, women are advised to avoid exercise in the supine position (lying on the back), because it decreases cardiac function. Adjust stretching and strength workouts accordingly.

• Eat enough to cover the demands of both pregnancy *and* exercise. For pregnancy alone, an extra 150 calories per day is recommended in the first two trimesters, and an additional 300 calories per day in the final trimester. And for running, figure an additional 100 calories for each mile you cover.

• As your belly grows, consider running with a maternity belt, an adjustable elastic band that straps around your hips and helps support the weight of your midsection.

WHEN TO NOT RUN

The American College of Obstetrics and Gynecology offers the following guidelines for curtailing exercise. Some pregnant women who exhibit the following risk factors might be advised to limit or not engage in exercise.

- Pregnancy-induced high blood pressure
- Preterm rupture of membranes (broken water)
- Premature dilation of the cervix or an incompetent cervix
- Preterm labor
- Second- or third-trimester vaginal bleeding
- A history of miscarriage

As always, check with your own health-care provider for the appropriate course of action.

• Finally, run only when you are comfortable. Some women run throughout their entire pregnancy. Others run only up to the seventh or eighth month, preferring to walk thereafter. It's interesting to note, though, that some women who are not comfortable running earlier in their pregnancy find that they enjoy it when they try again later. You can always take a break for a week or two and then try again to see if it feels better.

• For more information on this topic, the *Runner's World Guide to Running and Pregnancy* is a good resource.

POSTPARTUM RUNNING

Returning to exercise after labor and delivery can be, to put it mildly, a challenge. Some women report difficulty adjusting to their "new" bodies. It might take weeks or months before you feel able to exercise with regularity or intensity. Most women say it's several months at least—and more like 6 months or even a year—before they feel like their old selves again.

Of course, everyone has heard of women who feel perky enough to jump out of bed and run the day after they've given birth. But these women are the exception, and it's important never to feel rushed or pressured to return to fitness rapidly based on their example.

For the first few days after childbirth, focus on healing and resting. But even months afterward, your body is still slowly reverting to "normal" after changes that took place during pregnancy. "During pregnancy, there are a lot of stresses on the body due to changes in hormones and weight and posture. And with birth, it all changes again," Dr. Wells says. "The microarchitecture of the body has changed." That means you might be particularly prone to overuse injuries when you resume a running program after giving birth. The changes in your body are compounded by the fact that you're probably also deconditioned. And new stresses are involved too, not the least of which are lack of sleep and caring for the newborn baby.

"Going back slowly is the key," Dr. Wells says. Take extra care to listen to your body at this time, since many of the messages you'll receive will be new and unfamiliar. In particular, women who were avid runners before might "resume with a vengeance, maybe before the body is ready to take it on," she says.

Most important is understanding that neither your body nor your life will be the same after childbirth. The focus and intensity of your running will necessarily be different. For many women, fitting in exercise is a greater challenge once they have children. But it also can provide solace and release like never before.

Finally, be alert for real changes in your health, since pregnancy sometimes brings with it other health conditions. Excessive fatigue can be a sign of true complications, particularly a thyroid imbalance or anemia. If you feel endlessly tired, are unable to exercise at all, or find dramatic changes in your heart rate or appetite, be sure to check with a physician.

What You Can Do

Any exercise routine after childbirth should focus on health and well-being, rather than an immediate return to maximum fitness. Here's a suggested guideline for mothers who have had healthy, vaginal deliveries.

- **First few days.** Focus on rest and recovery.

- **First few weeks.** Begin exercise gradually and according to the way your body feels. In general, if you are not experiencing pain or excessive bleeding, light exercise is okay. For most women, this means beginning with walking and light stretching and calisthenics.

Focus on getting some alone time away from the baby, not dramatic fitness gains or weight loss. Stay well-hydrated, particularly if you are nursing.

• **After 6 weeks.** If your doctor gives the okay after your 6-week postpartum examination, you can begin gradually to resume your typical level of exercise. Proper hydration, nutrition, and rest are more important than ever.

You should return to running as if you were virtually new to the sport, beginning by alternating walking and jogging. This will allow you to respond to aches and pains and give the body's muscles, joints, bones, and connective tissue a chance to condition without injury. Follow all the general rules outlined earlier in chapter 2—increasing distance and intensity gradually and one at a time—to avoid getting hurt.

14

THE OLDER RUNNER

LONG MAY YOU RUN

To see how beneficial running is for us as we age, just look at some of the old masters of the sport lined up at the start of any race. Men and women into their sixties, seventies, and beyond are training and racing—and disproving plenty of myths about aging along the way.

"Most of aging is not due to age at all but rather to disuse," says Walter Bortz, M.D., a geriatrics specialist and professor of medicine at Stanford University for 30 years. In 2002, Dr. Bortz and his wife, Ruth Anne, made history as the oldest couple—both over the age of 70—to complete the Boston Marathon. Dr. Bortz shrugs off that accomplishment as if it were a mere warm-up, however. "My wife and I do 100-milers—it shows what the human body can do."

In fact, the aging human body is much more resilient than once believed. Senior runners have proven that the old chestnut "use it or lose it" is not just a saying but a fact. Research shows that exercising your muscles, heart, and lungs can stave off many of the ill effects and disease that typically accompany aging.

Doctors and scientists have long known that aerobic exercise lowers mortality rates; what hasn't been certain is whether intense exercise such as running can improve quality of life. The fear was that vigorous activity could accelerate the development of osteoarthritis, thus contributing to general disability for seniors.

A landmark 8-year study that followed hundreds of runners disproved this notion. The conclusions, reported in the mid 1990s, showed that the rate of development of disability was in fact several times lower in the runners than in a control group. The runners did not develop arthritis any faster, and they showed superior aerobic conditioning, bone density, organ functioning, and muscle strength. Over the 8 years, the runners showed a strikingly lower rate of disability—about a quarter of that of the sedentary group. They also exhibited lower body mass, experienced less joint pain and dysfunction, required fewer medications, and had fewer medical problems in general.

In short, exercise makes life better and more enjoyable for the elderly population. It makes what we ordinarily think of as the side effects of aging—muscle atrophy, aerobic declines, heavy reliance on medication, even depressed mental and emotional states—a dated concept, something that's not at all a given.

SPECIAL CONCERNS FOR THE AGING BODY

Running can reverse many of the effects of aging, but it can't stop time altogether. Some inexorable changes in the aging body make it more fragile and susceptible to injury. By taking commonsense precautions against common problems, older runners can lower their risk and remain healthy while training.

Dehydration. As we grow older, our ability to sweat and dissipate heat decreases. At the same time, the body's mechanism for indicating thirst grows increasingly unreliable with age. Chronic low-level dehydration is common in the older population, and it raises the risk of heat illness and compromised organ function and tissue strength. Running, of course, increases fluid requirements and can exacerbate the dehydration issue.

What you can do. It's very important for older runners to drink before and after exercise. While many younger runners can easily get through an hour-long workout without drinking, older runners should probably go no longer than 20 minutes to half an hour without drinking. Unlike young runners, who can safely rely on thirst as a guide to drinking, older runners should strive to consume 15 to 25 ounces of fluid per hour of exercise. A sports drink is preferable to plain water, since it replenishes electrolytes. Also, the flavor encourages you to drink more than if it were plain water.

Decreased flexibility. As we age, connective tissue loses its elasticity. This makes runners more susceptible to acute strains, pulls, and tears in muscles, tendons, and ligaments. Also, decreased range of motion results in a shorter, shuffling stride. Such biomechanical changes due to inflexibility increase the likelihood of overuse injury.

What you can do. Stretch. Inactivity only compounds tightness and loss of range of motion. Running helps to a certain degree, because it exercises the joints, but running also has an overall tightening effect on the body. That means stretching is the answer. One study of masters runners showed conclusively that 20 minutes of stretching three times a week significantly reduced inflexibility.

So even if you've ignored your stretching for years as a runner, now's the time to start. Supplement your training by stretching after every run, or at least three times a week. To ensure it gets done, factor stretching in to your total workout time, leaving at least 10 to 15 minutes after your run. Don't stretch before running, when the body is tight and inflexible. Muscles and joints are more limber after warming up on the run, which means you are less likely to strain something. Stretch all parts of your body—the legs and hips in particular. Be gentle and do not force a stretch or hold it too long. (See chapter 4 for the best stretches for runners.)

Loss of strength. Left to its own sedentary devices, the body loses muscle mass rapidly as it ages, typically by about 10 percent per decade beginning as early as our thirties or forties. (To make matters worse, muscle is generally replaced by additional adipose tissue, also known as fat.) The resulting loss in strength can be disastrous. Dr. Bortz points out that the number one predictor of whether you will require assistance as you age is leg strength. "It's not disease, not illness, but whether you have the strength to get in and out of a chair," he says.

What you can do. Running is one step toward battling the weakness that can come with age, but even running alone is not the best answer. To retain strength in all parts of the body, older runners should engage in a strength-training program that targets the whole body. Weight machines, available at any health club, are a great choice for an efficient, controlled workout. (Refer to chapter 5 for more on strength training.)

The amount of weight you lift needn't be heavy. It's more important to be consistent, working out two or three times a week and doing at least 10 to 12 repetitions of each exercise. If you want an individualized workout, your local recreational center or athletic club can help you find a trainer who specializes in geriatric conditioning. Trainers can be certified by several different organizations, the most reputable being the American College of Sports Medicine (ACSM) and the American Council on Exercise. Look for a trainer with a degree in exercise science or a health-related field, such as kinesiology. The ACSM Web site can help you find a trainer in your area with its ProFinder feature; go to www.acsm.org. Ask for references and check certifications.

Bone and joint health. Bone mass peaks when we're in our early thirties and generally slides downhill after that—the rate of which depends on many factors, including diet, genetics, and hormone levels. Bone density declines precipitously in many postmenopausal women, due to the lack of the female hormone estrogen, which both aids in the body's absorption of calcium and slows loss of calcium from bones.

Weak bones are more vulnerable to fractures. Compounding matters, broken bones are more serious for the elderly than for the young. Healing takes longer, and the resulting inactivity can take a toll in other areas, setting off a chain of disabilities. As we age, cartilage also tends to deteriorate. This makes joints vulnerable to injury and places them at greater risk of osteoarthritis.

It's a falsehood, long since disproved, that running damages bones or joints or hastens osteoarthritis. In fact, running protects against the decline of bone mass, fending off osteoporosis. And it's now believed that running might have a protective effect on the joints, as well.

What you can do. Weight-bearing exercise such as running is one of the best ways to maintain bone strength. That's because bone—just like muscle—responds to the demands you place on it with a conditioning response, toughening and hardening in reaction to stress. If you're a longtime runner, chances are your bones are now healthier for it. And if you're adhering to a strength-training program, it will pay double dividends since it also counts as a weight-bearing activity, thus providing a protective effect on bone density.

Beyond exercise, the most important way to protect bones is to eat a diet of healthy foods that are high in calcium. Milk, cheese, yogurt, and other dairy products are the best sources. Tofu, dark leafy vegetables, and canned salmon and sardines are also excellent choices. For extra insur-

BONE HEALTH AND HORMONE REPLACEMENT

Women should note that hormone replacement therapy (HRT) is no longer considered a safe way to protect bone health. Various forms of HRT had been widely prescribed since the 1960s to relieve symptoms of menopause and to protect women against heart disease. Along the way, it also was determined that HRT helps to maintain bone mass.

New research shows that not only does HRT (a mix of progestin and estrogen) *not* protect against heart disease, it might even contribute to it. It also might significantly raise the risk of stroke and some cancers.

Because of the health risks now associated with hormone replacement, women are advised to discuss all the pros and cons with their doctors so they can make an informed choice. But the medical consensus is that bone health alone is not enough reason to prescribe hormones.

---

ance, you can drink juice that is fortified with calcium and take a daily supplement that contains calcium.

Balance problems. Balance is one thing that young runners never think about—it comes naturally. But for older runners, balance often becomes a concern. "Like everything else, with age it gets worse," Dr. Bortz says. Loss of balance is due to a combination of factors, among them decreased sensory perception (hearing and vision), decreased tactile sensation (sense of touch), diminishing strength, and increased reaction time. Since falls are a primary cause of injury in older runners, loss of balance isn't just an inconvenience but can result in serious sprains and broken bones.

On the subject of falling, Dr. Bortz points out a caveat. Just because older runners are more likely to fall doesn't mean they should stop running. "I say you need to fall, or you're staying in bed too much," he jokes. In other words, the benefits of activity far outweigh the risk of injury.

The 8-year study of runners mentioned earlier confirms Dr. Bortz's position: While runners did indeed suffer more fractures and short-term disability than the sedentary group, their overall rate of disability was only a quarter of that of the control group.

What you can do. Balance exercises can help retain your sense of proprioception—knowing where your body is and what it is doing. Simple exercises can maintain your sense of balance and build strength in the tiny muscles that help to control it. A doctor, physical therapist, or athletic trainer can recommend balance exercises appropriate for

RUNNING AND HEART DISEASE

Running does not make you immune to heart disease or heart attack. Yes, the typical profile of a heart-attack victim is an out-of-shape, overweight individual with high blood pressure and a cigarette in hand. But runners—even very good ones—have indeed been struck down by heart attack.

"Too many runners feel that exercise is a panacea," says Paul Thompson, M.D., a professor of medicine at the University of Connecticut School of Medicine in Farmington, who is renowned for his expertise on the relationship of exercise and cardiac risks. Indeed, research confirms that regular aerobic exercise can significantly lower some of the risk factors of heart disease, improving cholesterol levels and blood pressure and keeping body weight in check. But the flip side is that exercise can't do anything about your inherited risk factors. And during exertion, the risk of heart attack actually increases.

So there are two sides to the story. "Exercise lowers the overall risk, but while running, it increases risk," Dr. Thompson explains. That's why even fit individuals can suffer sudden heart attack during exercise. These cases provide rare but cautionary tales. "If you have symptoms that might be heart disease, don't ignore them," advises Dr. Thompson.

There's no magic age at which you should undergo a cardiac

your age and condition. These might involve the use of a wobble board or exercise ball, or they could be as simple as standing on one leg with your eyes closed.

Dr. Bortz also recommends regular hearing and vision examinations. Poor sensory perception contributes to balance problems but is also an issue in itself, since hearing and vision problems make you vulnerable to external factors. A dog rounding a corner, for example, or a car coming down the street is more dangerous when you can't see or hear it in time to react.

evaluation. In fact, reserving such testing for people beyond a certain age can lead younger candidates for heart disease to a false sense of security. Instead, assessing your own risk with a doctor who knows you and whom you trust is the key, Dr. Thompson says. Factors that predispose you to heart disease include:
• Evidence of a family history of heart disease
• High blood pressure
• High cholesterol
• Diabetes
• Overweight
• Smoking

And what if you do show signs of heart disease? You might need to adjust your running regimen. But each case is different, and you must discuss the specifics with your physician. You might be instructed to back off intense exertion—give up the competition and the speed workouts, for example. In more advanced cases of heart disease, the focus might shift away from exercise altogether and instead toward lowering cholesterol and blood pressure with medication.

In the end, the responsibility lies with you to communicate with your doctor and ensure that you are running safe and smart. When it comes to your heart, running can remain your best friend far into old age. Just don't think that it makes you invincible.

TRAINING STRATEGIES

You can still run—and run hard—as you age. There's no reason to stop training seriously or racing at any age. And the principles of training remain the same. In fact, they're more important than ever. As we age, listening to our bodies becomes the overriding secret to preventing training-related injury.

You will need to make a few adjustments for your aging body. The primary difference as we age is that it takes our bodies longer to recover. This effect is noticeable as early as our thirties but becomes more pronounced with each passing decade.

Here are some guidelines for healthy training.

Maintain intensity. A weekly dose of speedwork or tempo runs obviously will help you retain your speed. Working near the limit of your aerobic capacity also prevents age-related declines. Studies have shown that runners who do regular speed training can largely maintain their capacity to use oxygen, whereas less strenuous exercise (easy jogging, for example) does not have the same beneficial effect.

Take extra recovery if you need it. Particularly after harder runs, you might notice you're not bouncing back as quickly as you used to. You might need 2 or 3 easy days between hard runs, instead of the 1 day you used to take. Let your legs be your guide. If they still feel soggy and listless, run easy until they regain their pep. If this means doing just one hard workout a week instead of two, that's fine. In fact, some runners switch to a 10-day cycle (rather than planning training in terms of 7-day weeks)—this allows them to fit in a long run, a track workout, and a tempo run without skimping on rest.

Consider lowering overall mileage. As we age, reduced strength and range of motion result in a shorter stride length. That means older runners generally must take more steps to cover the same amount of miles. The total number of steps we take is one of the predictors of overuse injury. So it's a fair safety precaution to cut your mileage slightly. This shouldn't hurt your racing ability; as mentioned above, your body responds largely to faster workouts when it comes to maintaining your speed.

Cross-train. The goal here is to reduce impact and repetitive pounding. Engaging in a variety of activities helps your body maintain fitness while minimizing your risk of injury. This principle is the same for runners of all ages; it just becomes even more important as we age and our joints and resiliency deteriorate. Swimming and cycling are both good cross-training supplements to running, since they do not deliver any impact to the joints. (See chapter 6 for more on cross-training options.)

Stretch and strengthen. As discussed in the previous section, muscle deterioration and loss of flexibility are two side effects of aging when your body is sedentary. Both can contribute to injury, but luckily, both can be countered to a great degree with strength and flexibility programs. (See chapters 4 and 5 for more on stretching and strength training.)

Wear proper shoes. It's more important than ever to be sure you're wearing the right shoes, since your joints are more susceptible to pounding. Be aware that as you age, your footwear needs might change. A reduction in stride length from tight joints, decreased muscle support, or even a change in posture can reconfigure your gait, resulting in a need for greater cushioning or support. Plan to buy new shoes at least once every year.

INDEX

Boldface page references indicate photographs and illustrations. Underscored references indicate boxed text.

Medical help
    alternative choices
        acupressure, 126—27
        acupuncture, 124—29
        chiropractic, 129—32
        massage, 122—24
    for disordered eating, 182
    orthopedist, 101
    physical therapist, 101
    podiatrist, 100—101
    sports medicine physician, 100
    in treating injuries, 99—103
    types of, 100—101
Medications. See Anti-inflammatories in
        treating injuries; specific types
Menstrual cycle and running, 179—81
Midsole of shoe, 34—35
Mileage
    goal, good, 21
    increasing
        after injury, 104
        gradual, 18—20
        separately from intensity increases,
            21
    older runners and, 196
Milk, 171
Minerals, 25. See also Supplements; specific
        types
Mittens for cold weather, 92
Moderation in running, 12—13, 16
Mortality rates and aerobic exercise, 189
Mother Nature. See Weather
Motion-control shoes, 33—34
Muscle soreness, typical, 23, 152
Muscle strains and tears, 110—11, 176

N

Neck and posture, 10—11
Neuroma, 117
New Balance shoes, 39
New runners
    cross-training for, 27—28, 68, 70, 151
    frequency of running and, 150—51
    health checkup and, 146—47
    hot weather and, 154—55
    hydration and, 159
    listening to body and, 145, 151—52, 151
    marathon and, 156—59
    racing and, 154—55
    rest and, 150—51
    shoes for, 147—49
    slow running for, 150

speed and, 150, 158
    training for, 158
    walking and running combination for,
        149—50
    weight loss and, 156—57
Nike shoes, 39
Nonsteroidal anti-inflammatories
        (NSAIDs), 99. See also Anti-
        inflammatories in treating injuries
Nordic skiing, 77—78
Novice runners. See New runners
NSAIDs, 99. See also Anti-inflammatories
        in treating injuries
Nutrition
    antioxidants and, 26
    bone health and, 179
    calcium and, 25—26, 170—71
    carbohydrates and, 25
    dieting and, avoiding, 156
    disordered eating and, 181—83
    eating habits and, 156—57
    fats and, 25
    magnesium and, 179
    in preventing injuries, 25—26
    protein and, 25
    supplements and, 25—26
    vitamin C and, 179
    vitamin D and, 171, 179
    women runners and, 25—26, 179,
        181—83
    young runners and, 170—71
Nutritionist, 182

O

Obesity epidemic, 161
Obsession with running
    incidence of, 133
    problems of, 136—39
    professional help for, 137
    professional knowledge about, 135
    recognizing, 134—36
    symptoms of, 134
Older runners
    aging and, 189
    balance problems and, 193—95
    bone health and, 192—93
    cross-training for, 68, 70, 196—97
    dehydration and, 190—91
    flexibility and, 191
    heart disease and, 194—95
    hydration and, 190—91
    intensity and, 196

Sunglasses for sun protection, 83, 88
Sun protection, 83, 88
Sunscreen, 88
Supercompensation, 17
Supination, 34
Supplements
    calcium, 25–26, 115
    daily, 25
    iron, 25–26
    nutrition and, 25–26
    women runners and, 25–26
Surfaces
    impact of running and, 3
    in preventing injuries
        soft, 28–29, 157
        varying, 27
Surgery in treating
    compartment syndrome, 108
    iliotibial band syndrome, 109
    plantar fasciitis, 112
    tendinitis of the Achilles, 119
Swimming, 73, 76

T

Taping ankle, 106, 106
Team sports, 79
Tears, muscle, 110–11, 176
Tempo runs, 13
Tendinitis of the Achilles, 118–19
Terrain
    impact of running and, 3
    in preventing injuries
        soft surfaces, 28–29, 157
        varying, 27
Therapist, 182
Thirst and hydration, 86
"Tired legs," 12, 22
Trail shoes, 38
Training
    adapting to current fitness, 4
    consistency and, 158
    hard effort, alternating with rest,
        22–23
    hard vs. smart, 19
    moderation and, 12–13, 16
    for new runners, 158
    for older runners, 196–97
    planning vs. practice and, 158
    proper
        mileage, gradually increasing, 18–20
        mileage and intensity, separately
            increasing, 21

principles of, 15–16, 28
    stress, adapting to, 16–18
severe changes in, avoiding, 4
sleep patterns and, 26
stress-recovery principle of,
    16–18
warm-up, 24–25
warning of injury and, paying attention
    to, 23–24
for young runners, 169, 170
Training effect, 17
Treadmill tests, 11, 108
Treating injuries. See also Medical help;
    PRICE (protection, rest, ice,
    compression, elevation)
alternative treatment choices
    acupressure, 126–27
    acupuncture, 124–29
    chiropractic, 129–32
    massage, 122–24
    popularity of, 121–22
    treatment habit and, 130
ankle sprain, 106–7, 106
anti-inflammatories
    ankle sprain, 106
    caution about, 98–99
    iliotibial band syndrome, 109
    plantar fasciitis, 111
    runner's knee, 113
    shin splints, 114
    tendinitis of the Achilles, 118
    types of, 99
blisters, 116
compartment syndrome, 108
cortisone injection, 112
hammertoe, 117
icing
    iliotibial band syndrome, 109
    muscle strains and tears, 110
    in PRICE treatment, 96–98, 97
    runner's knee, 113
    shin splints, 114
    tendinitis of the Achilles, 118
iliotibial band syndrome, 109
massage
    iliotibial band syndrome, 109
    muscle strains and tears, 110
    tendinitis of the Achilles, 119
medical help, 99–103
muscle strains and tears, 110
neuroma, 117
pain on top of foot, 117
patient's role in, 102